Get Serious Fitness

Get Serious Get Fit!

Presents:

"HARDCORE FITNESS"

TRAINING DEVELOPED IN SOME OF AMERICA'S TOUGHEST PRISONS.

This book is one of the first available products from **Get Serious Fitness**. If you purchased this book directly from **Get Serious Fitness**, a portion of the proceeds will be donated to the following organizations:

- **The National Center for Missing and Exploited Children**

- **Shriners Hospitals**

For more information, or to order this book from **Get Serious Fitness,** go to:

www.Myspace.com/getseriousfitness

Check out the **HARDCORE FITNESS** companion **DVD!**

This **DVD** shows live footage of inmates performing workouts shown in this book, as well as some not included in this book.

For a sneak-peek of the DVD, go to MySpace.com/Get Serious Fitness

Another organization that deserves an Honorable Mention is The Prison Scholar Fund. Its purpose is to help convicted felons turn their lives around through education. The PSF provides funding for inmates to attend college. I myself am a recipient of a scholarship through this fund It has definitely helped me to turn my life around. This book is evidence of that.

To find out more go to:

www.prisonscholarfund.org

ISBN 0-7414-5049-6

Published by:

INFINITY
PUBLISHING.COM

1094 New DeHaven Street, Suite 100
West Conshohocken, PA 19428-2713
Info@buybooksontheweb.com
www.buybooksontheweb.com
Toll-free (877) BUY BOOK
Local Phone (610) 941-9999
Fax (610) 941-9959

Printed in the United States of America

Printed on Recycled Paper

Published November 2008

Thanks and Dedications

First of all, I would like to thank all of those who helped make this book possible:

My Mother (I love you), my wife J.L., Marc the Norwegian, Summer Anderson, Brian Snelson, Dolphy (Blue) Jordan, Ty Wilshusen, Ty's Mom, Mr. A. and Mrs. K. at education, and Armondo Reed for "helping me to accomplish my goals."

Second, thanks to all of those who stuck by me, believed in me, or who consider themselves my friends.

And, especially to DZSQ you are the most special of all I Love You!!!

This book is dedicated to all of those who doubted me, and to the system that is designed to keep things like this from happening. Thank you for the motivation that drives me every single day!!!

Disclaimer:

The exercises, drills, circuits, and routines contained in this book are intended to give an inside look at some of the workouts done by prisoners. The descriptions serve as an illustration and are not intended as instructions. Any attempt to perform any of the exercises, drills, circuits, and/or routines contained herein is done at the individual's sole discretion. Attempting these exercises, drills, circuits, and/or routines is done at the individual's own risk.

As with any exercise regimen, consult your physician before beginning any exercise program.

Table of Contents

Introduction

The purpose of this book is to give an insider's look at some of the physical training that some inmates in America's prisons do. These exercises and workouts were developed in prisons where fancy equipment and special diets do not exist.

This book is the result of years of development. In the prison I have been writing this book there are very little resources available, so it took some time. However, I was unable to include everything that I wanted to, and polish it as much as I wanted to because the window of opportunity to make this book happen was very narrow. I am proud to say that I had absolutely no help from any editors or professionals; this book was written and formatted entirely by me. There were many obstacles that I had to deal with and patience definitely helped me to persevere. It was actually very much of a struggle to overcome the everyday bull that goes on in prison and to overcome the system that would prefer me to sit and do nothing with my time (believe it or not). It was my fight against a system, designed to keep people from aspiring to a higher level of living, that drove me to want to be more, to write this book, and start my own company from behind these walls.

Fitness became a passion of mine while incarcerated. One thing led to another, and I became a Certified Personal Trainer, got into school, and even started my own business. And this is only the beginning of many future plans that I have.

I decided to keep this book very simple and in laymen's terms so that any person should have little difficulty in understanding it. Occasionally I will do a little explaining and there are descriptions given for each exercise. These descriptions serve to paint a picture for readers and are not instructions on how to perform the exercises. I would like to have included photos of all of the exercises, but it just was not possible. The photos I did manage to get are not of the quality I would have liked either but I'm lucky to have gotten any photos at all.

As far as the exercises and routines described in this book, I myself have performed every single one, so I have not included anything that I have not done myself. I haven't necessarily invented everything in this book, although I do believe that I may be the first person who has done over 667 different kinds of push-ups (I'm not positive though). I have found these workouts to be very effective at improving the conditioning and performance of the body. I believe anyone could benefit from the exercises and workouts contained herein.

Fitness Inside

A stereotype exists for inmates in America's prisons. People usually associate prisoners with being in good physical condition and being tough. One might think, "no wonder the guys in prison are in good shape all they do is workout all day." Sometimes this is true, but not always. In many prisons weights have been removed, and there is minimal equipment available to use. Diets are poor at best, and recreational time and space is very limited. The prisons that have had weights removed and limited recreation times, are usually the prisons that have a problem with violence. But, in environments with a higher potential for violence, it is more important for individuals to remain in good physical condition, for obvious reasons. In my experience it was the inmates at these prisons who were in the best condition. There are several reasons for this.

For one thing, the whole atmosphere in these prisons is different. Violence can and does erupt on any given day without warning. Conditioning one's self in order to be prepared for these situations is taken much more serious as opposed to minimum custody prisons where a person doesn't have as much to worry about.

More importantly though, the inmates who are at prisons without weights and other equipment end up coming up with much better workouts. The reason for this is, as opposed to the inmates who have weights and usually focus more strictly on bodybuilding routines, which serve mostly to make an individual bigger and bulkier, these guys come up with workouts that improve overall conditioning and performance of the body.

The exercises and routines in this book were developed and are used in prisons where there was a complete lack of resources. These workouts work. These workouts can, beyond any doubt, improve the conditioning of any individual from beginner to elite athlete. These workouts:

- Are perfect for when there is little time available to workout.

- Are perfect for when there is no equipment available.

- Will work under any condition.

- Can be done any time, anywhere, as they have been done for years in cells the size of the average household bathroom.

Some professionals in the fitness industry have recently been marketing certain bodyweight routines as the latest and new best thing around. These workouts are nothing new; they are however, in my opinion, some of the best things around. These are not bodybuilding routines. They are full body performance routines. I myself have benefited greatly from using these workouts, and every single guy that I have trained using these workouts has seen marked improvements in fitness and performance levels, from beginner to bad-ass.

The workouts in this book do one thing. They give the biggest results in the shortest amount of time!

Breakdown

For ease of comprehension I have written this book in simple terms. I do not go into a lot of science or specifics, but instead try to paint a simple picture. The descriptions are just that, descriptions, and are not intended as instructions.

- **Single Exercises.** This section gives descriptions of over 80 exercises and 12 techniques for performing them.

- **Warm-up/Cool down.** This section explains in simple terms, the purpose and benefits of warming up and cooling down.

- **Jump Training.** This section gives descriptions of over 20 exercises used primarily to develop power.

- **667 Push-ups.** This section provides descriptions for hundreds of push-up variations.

- **Tumbling Drills.** This section provides descriptions for over 30 different drills used for a specialized conditioning.

- **Circuit Training.** This section describes circuit training, and provides some examples of circuits.

- **Hardcore.** This section gives descriptions of 5 high-intensity level routines.

Single Exercises

This section will show some of the many basic body weight exercises that inmates do. These single exercises are almost always used in circuit training (training using groups of exercises) that will be discussed in the Circuit Training section.

The exercises have been put into sections that are labeled as legs, core, etc. Although the exercises are categorized according to areas of the body, training using bodyweight exercises is not usually performed like training for bodybuilding (where certain areas of the body are trained at a time). These exercises are used to train the whole body to perform as a unit rather than exclusively training to make the muscles grow. I myself, on some days, train for strength, some days I train for power, and some days I train for endurance.

In addition to descriptions of the exercises themselves, there are a number of techniques that can be applied to most of the exercises. These techniques are listed first. I included different techniques for performing each exercise because each of these techniques serves a different purpose, and can actually alter the effects of the exercises. Some of the different purposes for the techniques are:

- **Variety**. Doing the same exercise the same way all of the time becomes boring, and therefore working out becomes boring. This leads to a lack of motivation to workout at all. Doing the same thing all of the time will also lead to what is known as a plateau in performance, that is, the body will cease to improve its performance levels beyond the workout it constantly receives.

- **Results**. Different movements, different angles of movement, different speeds of movement, and different rest periods, all have unique effects on the body. So by using these different techniques, even when performing the same exercise, the body is trained in different ways. For example, performing the squat exercise using the jump repetition technique will have a different effect on the body than performing the squat exercise using the 3-second repetition technique. The jump technique is good for improving explosiveness, whereas the 3-second repetition technique is good for improving endurance.

- **Quality**. When it comes to training, I believe in quality over quantity. One important factor in training the muscles is the amount of time that they are placed under tension. Many times when exercising, people perform the exercises incorrectly or hurriedly in order to complete more repetitions, mistakenly believing that because they counted higher, that they also performed better. More repetitions doesn't necessarily equate to a better workout. For example, when performing a push-up hurriedly for a set of twenty repetitions, each repetition would place the muscles under tension for approximately one second. The total amount of time that the muscles are under tension: 20 seconds. Compare this to a set of push-ups that are performed using the 3-second repetition technique for a set of only ten repetitions. Each of these repetitions will place the muscles under tension for approximately six seconds. Total time that the muscles are placed under tension using this technique: 60 seconds. Even though the person uses half of the number of repetitions, the time that the muscles are placed under tension is increased 3 times! Longer periods of tension means increased workload, which is one way of improving the quality of exercise.

For future reference:

• Concentric. Concentric movement or contraction means that the muscles shorten to flex. Example: During the push-up exercise, the upward motion is concentric. During the squat, the upward motion is concentric.

• Eccentric. Eccentric movement or contraction is the opposite of concentric movement or contraction. It is when the muscles lengthen while contracting. Example: When performing the push-up, the downward motion is eccentric. During the squat exercise the downward motion is eccentric as well.

• Isometric. Isometric contraction is when there is no movement of the muscles during contraction. They neither lengthen nor shorten while being flexed. Examples of isometric exercises are the Wall sit, the Plank, and the Bird dog.

• Strength. When training to improve strength levels using bodyweight exercises, resistance can be added. This is usually done with a partner.

• Power. When training to increase power using bodyweight exercises, Plyometrics, or Jump Training is used. (See Jump Training Section.)

• Endurance. Training to increase endurance using bodyweight exercises is done in a few different ways. The first is to increase the number of repetitions. The second is to use the repetition techniques that increase the time that the muscles are placed under tension such as the 3-second rep. technique. The third is to shorten rest periods between exercises.

Techniques for performing each repetition.

These techniques can be applied to most exercises listed in this book. These techniques for performing each repetition can also be combined with the techniques for performing each exercise to create even more possibilities. So that you understand what these techniques are for here are two examples:

Example #1 Rather than simply performing the Chin-up exercise as normal, perform the exercise using the 3-second repetition technique by lifting the body and lowering the body through the full range of motion three seconds up and three seconds down.

Example #2 Instead of performing the squat exercise as normal, perform the exercise using the 1¼ repetition technique. That is, coming up only a quarter of the way from the bottom during the concentric phase of the squat, lowering back to the bottom, and then completing a full repetition.

1.   Jump

The jump is performed by jumping completely off of the ground during the concentric phase of the exercise. Jumps are done quickly and explosively. For instance, when performing a squat as a jump, first lower the body toward the ground as in a normal squat, but then instead of raising the body as in a normal squat, explode upward to jump completely off of the ground. (Also see the Jump Training section)

Why? This technique helps to improve power and explosiveness.

2.   Negative Repetitions.

Negative repetitions are done by performing the eccentric phase of the exercise slowly, from 3 seconds to as long as one wishes. The concentric phase is performed at normal speed.

Why? This technique increases the time in which the muscles are placed under tension and therefore increases the workload of a given set. It can help to increase muscular endurance as well.

3.   3 Second Repetitions.

3-second repetitions are performed slowly on both the concentric and eccentric phases of the exercise. They are basically slow motion exercises performed at 3 seconds down and 3 seconds up.

Why? This technique increases the time in which the muscles are placed under tension and therefore increases the workload of a given set. It can help to improve muscular endurance as well.

4.   Top and Bottom Pause.

Using the top and bottom pause, the body is held and all muscles are flexed for a period of one full second or more at the very top and the very bottom of the range of motion of the exercise.

Why? This technique adds a brief isometric contraction at the top and bottom of the range of motion, which helps to increase the workload.

5.   1¼ Repetitions.

One of my favorites, one-and-a-quarter repetitions are done simply by performing a quarter of a repetition, followed by a full repetition. For example, when performing a push-up, first, lower the body completely, then come up only a quarter of the way, then lower completely, and finally, come up all of the way to the top.

Why? Performing 1¼ repetitions, (say ten reps), you not only get ten full repetitions, you also get ten quarter-repetitions that add strength and endurance to that specific shortened range of motion. This also increases the workload by increasing the amount of time that the muscles are placed under tension.

6.   1,2,3's.

1,2,3's are a variation of the 1¼ reps. The difference being that the first repetition comes up from the bottom of the range of motion only one third of the way up, the second repetition comes up even further to two-thirds of a full rep, and the third repetition is a full range rep or all of the way to the top.

Why? Performing 1,2,3's, you get the same added benefit of the 1¼ reps, but with even more added workload per repetition.

7.   Short Burns.

Short burns are performed by staying in a short range of motion within the full range of motion, and performing quick short repetitions. Example #1 when performing the squat exercise, come up only about one-third of the way on the concentric (upward phase) of the squat. Simply perform all of the repetitions in the bottom one-third of the range of motion. Example #2 when performing a pull-up let the chin drop only a few inches below the pull-up bar and keep the body in the upper third of the range of motion. Make sure not to allow the body to get all of the way to the top or bottom of the full range of motion, however, as this can give the muscles a rest and part of the reason for this technique is to keep them under constant tension.

Why? Short burns apply all of the workload to a specific range within the full range of motion and keep the muscles under constant tension.

Techniques for performing each set.

Apply these techniques to the exercises listed in the book. These techniques can also be combined with the repetitions techniques for even more possibilities. Here are two examples for a better understanding.

Example #1 Rather than performing a push-ups exercise as normal, use the forced reps technique to force yourself to complete two extra repetitions.

Example #2 Combine the negative repetitions technique listed previously, with the forced repetitions technique listed below while performing a set of push-ups. That is, perform the push-ups slowly during the eccentric phase, and when the set is complete, force two more push-ups.

1.   Super set.

A superset is performing two exercises back and forth. For example, first perform a set of push-ups, then, perform a set of squats, then rest. Repeat.

Why? Performing supersets makes more efficient use of workout time. See the Circuit Training Section for further details of how this works.

2.   Forced Repetitions.

Forced repetitions are done by performing a set to failure, and then forcing one's self to get one or two more reps either with a partner to assist or spot you, or by resting for just a couple of seconds before completing the two forced reps. I myself like to use these for performing pull-ups.

Why? Forced repetitions push the muscles farther than they're used to, thereby increasing the workload. In order to make gains in performance levels, it is necessary to, when the body is ready, push the body beyond what it is accustomed to. Otherwise, the body will become complacent and cease to improve its performance. Say you can do ten pull-ups but no more. When you force the body to do two more, after a short rest, pretty soon the body will adapt and you will be able to do twelve pull-ups.

3.   Ascending Repetitions.

Using this technique, one does a number of repetitions, stops briefly for a short rest, and then does a set of one more repetition than before. Example: Do three push-ups, stand, do four push-ups, stand, do five push-ups etc. The exercise that I have seen most commonly used with this technique is squats. It is called the walking 20. To perform, do one squat, then take 2-5 steps forward, then do two squats, etc. until twenty is reached. The total repetitions performed will be 210. Usually this can be done in around five minutes.

Why? Like forced reps, ascending repetitions help to push the body farther than it is accustomed to in a shorter time period.

4.   Descending Repetitions.

Descending repetitions are just the opposite of the ascending repetitions. They are performed by doing a certain number of repetitions, stopping to rest briefly, and then doing a set of one less repetition than before. Example: Do ten pull-ups; drop off of the bar for a few seconds, then do nine pull-ups, etc.

Why? Descending repetitions help to push the body farther than it is accustomed to, and are easier than ascending repetitions because one less rep is performed than before as opposed to one more than before.

5.   Circuits (See Circuit Training Section)

Single Body-Weight Exercises

For this book, I have tried to include mostly no-equipment body-weight exercises. Partners can be used in different ways to help add resistance etc. There are many variations of some exercises, although I have included only one or two for each.

The exercises are also placed into categories of intensity or difficulty. Level 1 being the easiest to perform, and Level 3 being the hardest to perform. For those who I have trained, the general rule was that the lower levels served as a pre-requisite to the higher levels. Meaning a person should be able to perform all of the lower levels without difficulty before attempting the higher levels.

Leg Exercises.

These exercises are used to increase lower body strength, power, and endurance.

LEVEL 1

❖ **Squat.**

➢ Start position: Standing upright, feet shoulder width apart.

➢ Squat straight down by bending at the knees until the legs are bent at a 90-degree angle.

➢ Stand back up into the start position.

➢ Repeat.

Weight can be added with a partner seated up on the shoulders.

❖ **Hip raise.**

➢ Start position: Lying on the back with the knees bent (in sit-up position.)

➢ Raise the hips up as high as possible by pushing with the feet against the ground, and return to start position.

➢ Repeat.

❖ **Hamstring reach.**

➢ Start position: Standing straight with feet shoulder width apart.

➢ Raise both hands overhead and take a large step forward with the right leg.

➢ Bend the right knee as little as possible while bringing the hands down to touch the ground in front of the right foot.

➢ Repeat with the left then right, back and forth.

❖ **Calve raise.**

Calve raises can be performed with or without a partner.

➢ Start standing feet shoulder width apart.

➢ Raise the body by lifting with the calves (standing up on the balls of the feet.) lower and repeat.

➢ Weight can be added with a partner seated up on the shoulders.

LEVEL 2

❖ **Split squat.**

➢ Start position: Standing upright with the feet shoulder-width apart.

➢ Take one step forward with the right foot so that the feet are split apart.

➢ From this position, perform the squat exercise.

➢ For the next set, the foot positions are reversed.

❖ **Tiptoe squat.**

➢ Start position: Start by standing on the balls of the feet (heels off of the ground) with the feet no more than 2 inches apart.

➢   Keeping the feet close together, and staying on the balls of the feet, perform the squat exercise.

❖   Lunge.

This exercise is similar to the split squat except that the feet are split farther apart.

➢   Start position: Standing upright with feet shoulder-width apart.

➢   Take one large step forward with the right foot and lower the body by bending the right knee to a 90-degree angle.

➢   Step back into the starting position. For the next set, step with the left foot.

➢   Repeat

Lunges can also be done by stepping with only one foot at a time rather than alternating back and forth, or taking steps forward and/or backward lunging along the way.

❖   Step-ups.

➢   Start position: Start by standing upright in front of a box or other elevated surface.

➢   Step up with the right foot onto the box and then step back down.

➢   Step up with left foot onto the box and then back down.

➢   Repeat for desired number of reps or time period.

These can also be done one foot at a time (step up with the right foot only for 20 reps for example.)

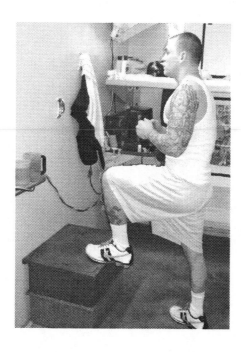

❖ **Side to side.**

➢ Start position: Stand straight up with feet wide apart and toes pointed straight forward.

➢ The body is shifted first to the left, bending the left knee but keeping the toes pointed forward, then to the right, back and forth.

(Almost as if lunging sideways but both feet remain in the start position and do not leave the ground)

❖ **Run stairs.**

➢ Start position: Start standing at the bottom of a staircase.

➢ Run up to the top of the staircase and back down again.

➢ Repeat for designated time period or number of reps.

❖ **Duck walk.**

➢ Start position: Standing upright with the feet shoulder width apart, squat down to the bottom of the squat position. Both knees are bent to 90 degrees and the hands are placed out in front of the face or on top of the head. Walk forward or backward in this position.

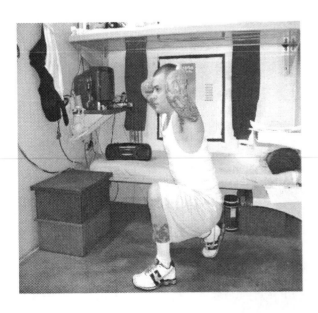 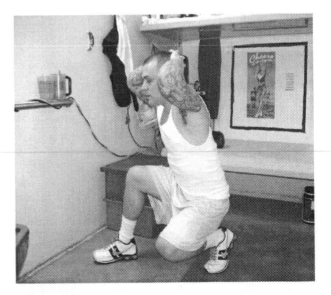

❖ **Wall-sit.**

➢ Start position: Start with the back against a wall in the bottom of the squat position and hands at the sides.

➢ Hold for as long as possible, or for a designated time, keeping the back flat against the wall and the knees bent in a 90-degree angle. Do not use the hands to help hold the position.

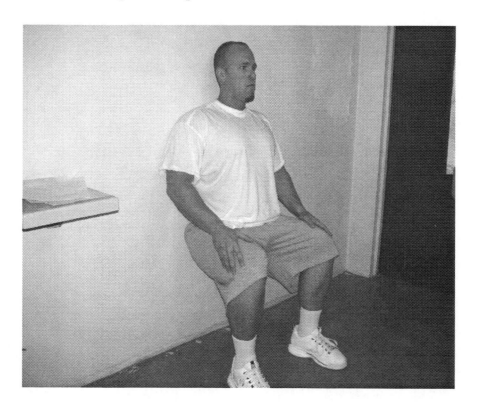

LEVEL 3

❖ **High-knee run.**

➢ Start position: Start by standing upright feet shoulder width apart.

➢ Stepping as high as possible with each knee, run forward. This is not a fast run, but instead, the knees are to be lifted explosively, as high as possible and toward the chest with each step.

These can also be done by placing the hands against a wall and pushing against the wall while stepping.

❖ **One leg squat.**

➤ Start position: Standing upright, feet shoulder width apart.

➤ Lift the right leg straight out in front of the body while putting the hands out in front of the body or to the sides to maintain balance.

➤ Squat down with the left leg, and then stand.

➤ Repeat on both sides.

❖ **Walking piggyback squat. (Requires a partner)**

➤ Start position: Partner A stands upright and partner B climbs up onto partner A's back in a piggyback position.

➤ Partner A then takes 2 steps forward with partner B on his back.

➤ Once he has taken 2 steps forward, he performs a designated number of squats (usually 1 or 2.)

➤ This is repeated until a certain distance has been covered or a designated number of squats have been reached.

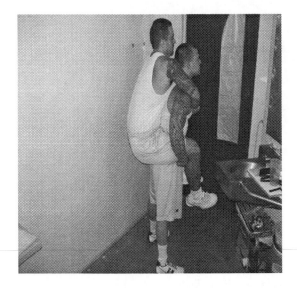 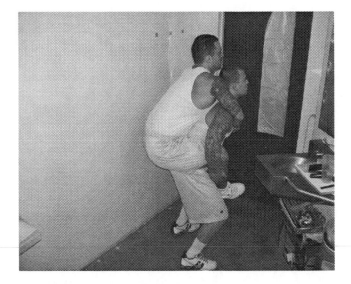

❖ **Hamstring drop. (Requires a partner)**

This is a very difficult exercise and is definitely not recommended for beginners.

➤ Start position: Partner A starts upright and on his knees, partner B is behind him to hold his ankles, keeping his feet from coming off of the ground.

> Keeping his body rigid and straight, partner A then lowers himself to the ground by extending (straightening) the knees.

> Once he reaches the ground he raises himself back to the starting position using his hamstring muscles to lift him.

> Repeat.

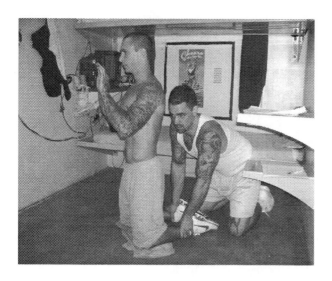 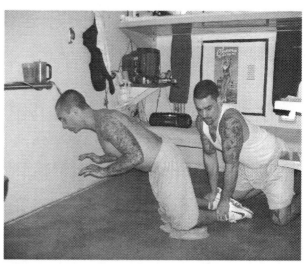

❖ **Quick step-ups.**

> Start position: Standing in front of box or some other elevated surface (the box should not be higher than 18 inches.)

> Step up with the right, then left foot, and then back down as fast as possible. This exercise is to be performed very quickly.

> Repeat for specific time period or number of reps.

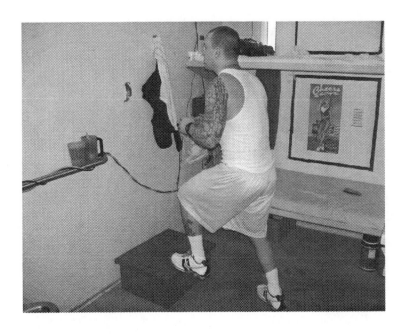

❖ Pick-ups. (Requires a partner)

➤ Start position: Partner A stands directly behind partner B.

➤ Partner A then squats down, grabbing partner B around the waist or thighs.

➤ Partner A lifts partner B using the legs to lift. He then sets him back down.

➤ Repeat.

There are many ways to perform pick-ups this is just one example.

❖ Leg-Drives. (Requires a partner)

➤ Start position: Partner A stands facing partner B.

➤ Partner A then drives forward into partner B placing his shoulder against partner B's mid-section, and pushing with the legs.

➤ He continues to drive forward for a certain distance or time period, while partner B attempts to keep him from moving forward or at least adds resistance to his progress.

➤ Partners switch positions and repeat.

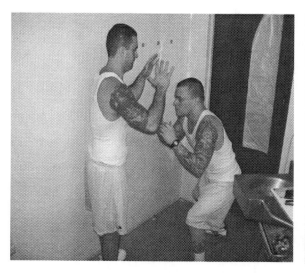 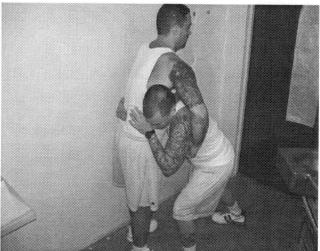

❖ **Jumps. (See Jump Training section)**

Core Exercises

These exercises are used to increase the strength, power, and endurance of the core (mid-section).

LEVEL 1

❖ **Sit-up.**

➢ Start position: Lying on the back with the knees bent. The feet are placed close together and close to the buttocks. The hands are placed on the temples or with fingertips on the ears, not behind the head.

➢ Sit-up while keeping the feet on the ground and in the same position. Return to start position.

➢ Repeat.

❖ **Crunch.**

➢ Start position: Lying flat on the back with the feet lifted up off of the ground, and the knees bent at a 90 degree angle so that the upper legs point straight up and the lower legs are parallel to the ground. The hands are placed on the temples or fingertips to the ears, not behind the head or neck. The feet may be held in the air or placed on a raised surface.

➢ Crunch the abs by bringing the sternum toward the pelvis. Hold at the top briefly, and then lower.

➢ Repeat.

❖ **Ankle reach.**

➢ Start position: Sit-up position but with the hands at the sides.

➢ One at a time, reach down and touch each ankle. Start by reaching with the right hand down to touch the right ankle, and then reach with the left hand to touch the left ankle.

➢ Crunch and flex the abs and oblique muscles throughout the entire range of motion.

➢ Repeat.

❖ **Windmill.**

➢ Start position: Standing straight with feet wider than shoulder width and hands extended straight out to the sides at shoulder height.

➢ Reach down with the left hand and touch the right foot.

➢ Return to the start position, and reach down with the right hand to the left foot.

➢ Repeat back and forth.

❖ **Toe Touch (standing).**

➢ Start position: Standing straight feet shoulder width apart hands above the head and pointed straight up.

➢ Bend down at the hip and touch the toes with the hands. Return to start position and repeat.

LEVEL 2

❖ **Crossover sit-up.**

➢   Start position: Same as sit-up position.

➢   Instead of sitting straight up as with the sit-up, the torso is twisted while sitting up so that the left elbow crosses over to touch the right knee.

➢   Repeat back and forth with the left elbow to the right knee, and the right elbow to the left knee.

❖ **Half sit-up.**

➢   Start position: Same as sit-up position but with the hands placed on the hips.

➢   Sit-up crunching the sternum to the pelvis and hold at the top.

➢   Repeat.

❖ **Hands under sit-up.**

➢   Start position: Same as the sit-up position, but the hands are placed beneath the small of the back. The hands should not be placed below the buttocks.

➢   Sit-up by crunching the sternum toward the pelvis and hold at the top for one full second. The hands should remain flat against the ground.

➢   Repeat.

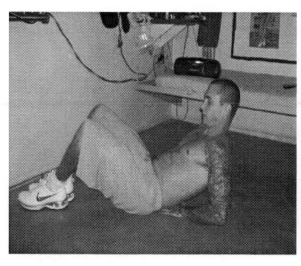 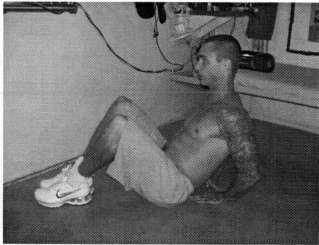

❖ **Sit-up Hip-up.**

This exercise is a combination of the hip raise (leg exercises) and sit-up exercises.

➢ Start in the sit-up position.

➢ First, perform a sit-up.

➢ Then, perform a hip raise as described in the Leg Exercises section.

➢ Repeat.

❖ **Hands under crunch.**

➢ Start position: Crunch position, but with hands placed under the small of the back with palms flat against the ground.

➢ The crunch is performed the same as the regular crunch.

➢ Repeat.

❖ **Crossover crunch.**

➢ Start position: Crunch position.

➢ Rather than simply crunching the sternum to the pelvis, twist the torso while crunching and bring the left elbow toward the right knee, and then the right elbow to the left knee.

❖ **Twisting side crunch.**

➢ Start position: Same as the sit-up. Start by lying the left leg down on the ground so that the outer thigh is flat against the ground, leave the right leg up in start position but slightly closer to the left leg.

➢ Crunch sideways rather than the normal way by bringing the right elbow to the right knee.

➢ Switch sides and repeat.

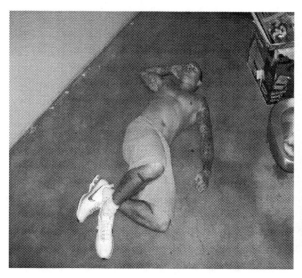 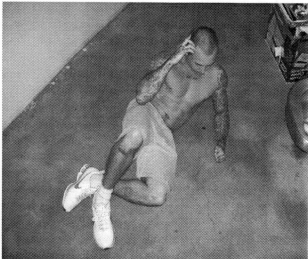

❖ **Reverse crunch.**

➢ Start position: Lying flat on the back and arms at the sides.

➢ Bring the legs up while bending at the knee. Continue this motion and lift the hips off of the ground until the knees touch the chest.

➢ The crunching of the abs is the same as in the crunch, but in reverse. (The pelvis is brought toward the sternum rather than the sternum brought toward the pelvis.)

❖ **Knee-up (sitting).**

➢ Start position: Sitting on a bench or on the ground balanced on the buttocks, with the feet lifted a couple inches from the ground. The hands are placed at the sides to keep balanced.

➢ Bring the knees to the chest and squeeze the abs. Like the reverse crunch, the pelvis is being crunched toward the sternum.

➢ The legs are then extended back to the start position.

➢ Repeat. To add difficulty, place hands on the temples instead of at the sides.

❖ **Toe touch (lying).**

➢ Start position: Lying on the back, flat on the ground, with the hands to the sides.

➢ Raise the feet to a height of about two or three feet from the ground, while keeping the legs straight and together.

> Reach up and touch the toes; keeping the legs straight out. Crunch the abs while doing this.

> Repeat.

❖ One leg twist.

> Start position: Lying on the back, flat on the ground. Bend the right knee so that the right leg is in a position similar to the sit-up position. Extend the left arm straight out to the side for balance. Place the right hand on the right temple.

> Simultaneously lift the left leg; keeping the knee unbent, while lifting the upper body and twisting so that the right elbow touches the left knee.

> Lower and repeat.

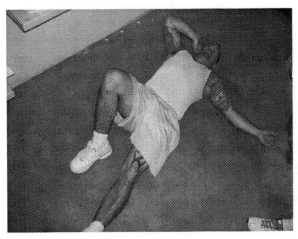 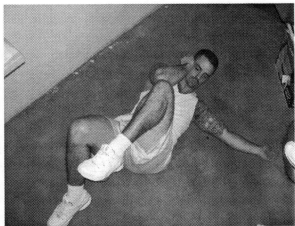

❖ Leg raise (lying).

> Start position: Lying flat on the back on the ground.
> Keeping the legs straight, lift them between six and twenty-four inches off of the ground.
> Lower the legs to start position and repeat.

❖ Cutting edge.

This exercise is similar to the leg raise exercise except for that when the legs are at the top of the raise, say eighteen inches off of the ground, the legs are separated so that the individual is basically doing the splits in the air.

> Start position: Same as the leg raise.

➤ Bring the legs up off of the ground, split them apart in the elevated position, put them back together, and lower the legs.

➤ Repeat.

❖ **Flutter kick.**

➤ Start position: Same as the leg raise. Instead of lifting the legs together, one leg is lifted at a time.

➤ Start with both legs about six inches from the ground.

➤ First lift the left leg to about eighteen inches and lower to start position, then bring the right leg up and lower back to start position.

➤ Repeat, never lowering the legs below six inches above the ground.

❖ **Bicycle.**

➤ Start position: Crunch position.

➤ This exercise is done by first bringing the right knee to the left elbow, and then the left knee to the right elbow. The feet are moved in a fashion similar to peddling a bicycle (hence the name of the exercise). The torso is twisted to bring each elbow to each knee back and forth while "peddling" with the feet.

❖ **Side leg raise (lying).**

➤ Start position: Lying flat on the side, on the ground.

➤ If starting lying on the left side, extend the left arm out for balance, and put the right hand against the temple. Lift the right leg, keeping the knee straight, and at the same time, bring the right elbow up to touch the right knee. Flex the oblique muscles at the top.

➤ Switch sides and repeat.

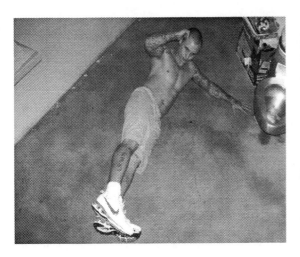 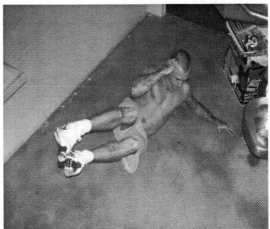

❖ Knee-up (standing).

➢ Start position: Standing straight with the feet shoulder width apart, and the hands on the temples.

➢ One at a time, bring the each knee up toward the chest, while bringing the elbow down to meet the knee, left knee to right elbow, and right knee to left elbow.

This exercise is kind of like performing a standing bicycle exercise.

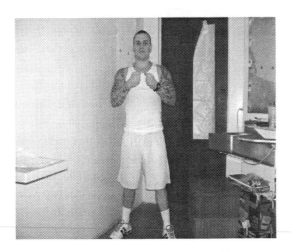 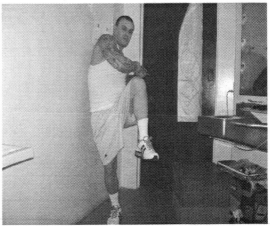

❖ Side bends.

➢ Start position: Standing straight feet shoulder width apart and hands on the temples.

➢ Bend down sideways at the hip and bring the left elbow to the left thigh, then bend to the other side bringing the right elbow to the right thigh.

➢ This can also be done with the hands held high above the head. Instead of bringing the elbow to the thigh, simply bend down sideways as far as possible on each side.

These can also be done one side at a time.

❖ Plank.

➢ Start position: Start in a position similar to the push-up position except that the forearms are placed flat on the ground to hold up the body instead of the hands. The feet are placed together with the toes on the ground and the body in a straight line, meaning that if a broomstick is placed on the back, the stick should touch the head, the upper back, the buttocks and the calves.

➢ Hold this position as long as possible or for predetermined time periods.

❖ Side plank.

This exercise is the same as the plank except for that it is done on the side.

➢ Start position: Feet together, the left foot is sideways against the ground and the body is held up in a straight line on the left forearm. The right arm rests against the right side. This position can be easily reached starting from the plank position and then rolling on to one side.

➢ Hold this position for as long as possible or for predetermined time periods.

➢ Switch sides and repeat.

❖ Bird dog.

➢ Start position: Start with both hands and knees on the ground.

➢ Reach up and point straight out with the right hand, while lifting the left leg up and behind the body, the knee unbent. Hold for a predetermined amount of time before switching to the left hand and right leg.

➢ Repeat.

❖ Superman.

➢ Start position: Lying flat on the stomach with the hands in front of the head and pointed forward (like Superman flying through the air.)

➤ Bring the hands up off of the ground and as high as possible, while simultaneously bringing the feet off of the ground as high as possible.

➤ Hold for as long as possible or for a predetermined amount of time by flexing the lower back muscles. These can be done by holding briefly, and repeating instead of holding for as long as possible.

➤ Return to the start position and repeat.

LEVEL 3

❖ **Sit-up stand-up. (Requires a partner)**

➤ Start position: Partner A starts in the sit-up position with partner B holding his ankles, securing his feet to the ground.

➤ Partner A performs a sit-up, and at the top of the sit-up exercise, he stands straight up.

➤ Partner A then squats all of the way back down to the top of the sit-up position.

➤ Repeat.

❖ **Pike.**

➤ Start position: Lying flat on the back with hands straight above the head.

➤ Rather than lifting the legs and then reaching up with the upper body, as with the lying toe touch, lift both the legs and the upper body simultaneously and touch the toes at the halfway point.

➤ Lower the legs and upper body to the start position and repeat.

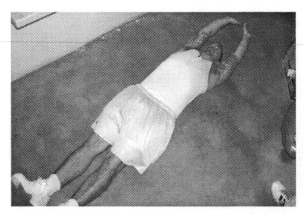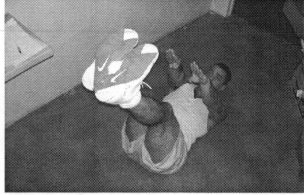

❖ **Leg raise (hanging).**

➤ Start position: Hanging from a pull-up bar or other type of elevated bar.

➤ Bring the legs straight up as high as they will go, while keeping the knees unbent and the legs held together.

➤ Make sure not to swing the legs up, but make this exercise count by controlling the speed at which the legs are raised.

➤ Lower and repeat.

❖ **Knee-up (hanging).**

➤ Start position: Hanging from a pull-up bar or other type of elevated bar.

➤ Bring the knees to the chest as in the Knee-up (sitting) exercise. Again, take care not to swing the legs.

➤ Lower and repeat.

Shoulder Exercises

These exercises are used to increase the strength, power, and endurance of the shoulders. Shoulders are definitely the hardest muscle group to train without using equipment.

LEVEL 1

❖ **Circles.**

➤ Start position: Standing straight with the feet shoulder width apart and the arms extended out to the sides at shoulder height.

➤ Move the arms in a forward circular motion for designated time or number of circles.

➤ Move arms in a backward circular motion.

➤ The arms can also be placed out in front of the body or above the head. The circular motion can be large or small.

LEVEL 2

❖ **Push-ups. (See push-ups section)**

❖ **Bear crawl.**

➢ Start position: Start on all fours (hands and feet on the ground.)

➢ Crawl forward, backward, or even sideways, with the hands and feet. (Backwards works the shoulders best.)

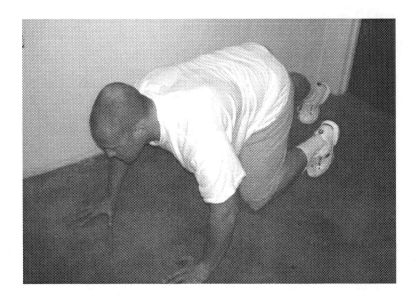

LEVEL 3

❖ **Handstand shoulder press.**

➢ Start position: Standing on the hands, with a partner holding the feet in the air. Without a partner, the feet are placed against a wall.

➢ Standing on the hands, lower the body toward the ground until the top of the head or the nose touches the ground.

➢ Push back up to the start position and repeat.

❖ **Wheelbarrow walk. (Requires a partner)**

➢ Start position: Start in push-up position but with partner A holding partner B's feet up off of the ground (like handles of a wheelbarrow.)

> Partner B then crawls forward or backward on the hands while partner A holds the feet.

(Handstand Shoulder press.)

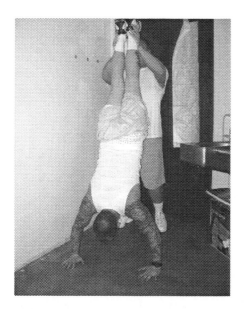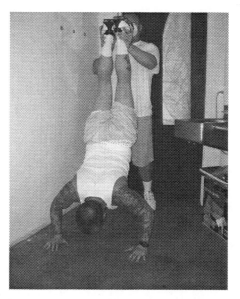

Back Exercises

These exercises are used to increase the strength, power, and endurance of the back muscles.

LEVEL 1

❖ **Toe touch (standing) (See Core Exercises)**

LEVEL 2

❖ **Superman. (See Core Exercises)**

❖ **Plank. (See Core Exercises)**

❖ **Back extensions.**

> Start position: Using a Roman chair or back extension platform.

➤   Start by lowering the body as far as it will reach.

➤   Now bring the body back up by extending (straightening) the lower back.

➤   Repeat.

❖   **Pull-ups.**

➤   Start position: Hanging from a pull-up bar with a pronated (palms facing away from the body) grip.

➤   Pull the body up until the chin is raised above the bar.

➤   Lower to start position.

➤   Repeat.

❖   **Chin-ups.**

➤   Start position: Hanging from a pull-up bar with a supinated (palms facing the body) grip.

➤   Lift the body until the chin is raised above the bar.

➤   Lower to start position.

➤   Repeat.

LEVEL 3

❖   **Plyometric pull-ups.**

Instead of simply performing the normal pull-up, this pull-up is performed explosively.

➤   Start position: Pull-up position.

➤   From the start position, explode upward and release the bar and clap the hands together at the top of the motion.

➤   Catch the bar on the downward motion and repeat immediately.

❖   **Around the world pull-ups.**

➤   Start position: Pull-up position.

➤ Instead of pulling straight up, pull up in a circular motion and to the right so that the chin is above the right hand on the bar.

➤ Keeping the chin above the bar, continue the circular motion so that the chin is above the left hand before lowering to the start position.

➤ Repeat in the opposite direction.

❖ **Side to side pull-ups.**

These are similar to the around the world pull-ups.

➤ Start position: Pull-up position.

➤ Pull-up so that the chin is above the bar.

➤ Keeping the chin above the bar, shift so that the chin is above the right hand, and then move the other direction until the chin is above the left hand.

➤ Repeat back and forth from side to side for a designated number of times, then lower to the start position and repeat.

❖ **Pull-up V's.**

➤ Start position: Pull-up position, but with the legs held straight out in front of the body by flexing at the hips to a 90 degree angle.

➤ Perform pull-ups while holding the legs in the extended position.

❖ **Up and over pull-ups.**

These are done explosively.

➤ Start position: Pull-up position.

➤ Perform a pull-up and when at the top of the pull-up position, use the momentum to continue up over the bar, and finish with the arms fully extended, and completely above the bar. (As if hoping a fence).

➤ Repeat.

❖ **Two-Finger Pull-ups.**

➤ Start position: Pull-up position.

➤ Now, instead of hanging on as normal, switch the grip on the bar to only hanging on with the index and middle fingers.

➤   Perform pull-ups using this grip.

❖   **Back and forth Pull-ups.**

➤   Start position: Pull-up position.

➤   Start by performing one pull-up.

➤   Next, climb with the hands to the far left of the pull-up bar and perform another pull-up.

➤   Now, climb to the far right and perform yet another pull-up.

➤   Continue back and forth.

Arm Exercises

These exercises are used to increase the strength, power, and endurance of the arms. Although the exercises have more purpose than just to work the arms, they are great for arm exercises as well and are used to train arms.

LEVEL 1

❖   **Grips.**

➤   This exercise is to strengthen the hands and forearms. An object such as a racquetball is squeezed or a wet towel is twisted. Another kind of grip exercise is to start with the arms extended outward from the body to the sides. Make a fist fifty times as if squeezing an object, then bring the arms out in front of the body and repeat. Finally, put the arms straight up over the head and do fifty more.

LEVEL 2

❖ **Push-ups (See Push-ups Section)**

❖ **Bar dips.**

❖ **Triceps extension.**

➢ Start position: Using some elevated platform, the hands are placed upon the platform at about shoulder width.

➢ Lower the body by flexing the arms (bending at the elbows.) Make sure to keep the elbows tucked in close to the body throughout the exercise.

➢ When the arms reach a 90-degree angle at the elbow, lift the body back to the start position by extending the arms.

❖ **Pull-ups/chin-ups. (See Back Exercises)**

❖ **Crab Walk.**

➢ Start position: Start by sitting on the ground.

➢ Now lift the body off the ground, and onto the hands and feet.

➢ Crawl forward, backwards, or sideways in this position.

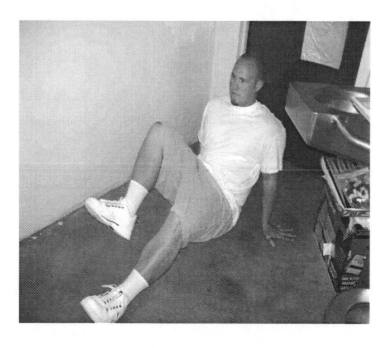

❖ **Bear crawls. (See Shoulder Exercises)**

❖ **Hanging grips.**

➢ (#1) Hang from pull-up bar as long as possible, or for a designated time period.

➢ (#2) Drape a towel or sheet over a pull-up bar and hang from it as long as possible, or for a designated time period.

➢ (#3) A sheet is hung over a pull-up bar, so that it is like a rope. It is then climbed up and down using only the hands and arms (let the lower body hang).

Chest Exercises

Use these exercise to increase the strength, power, and endurance of the chest muscles.

LEVEL 1

❖ **Isometric squeeze.**

➢ Start by standing or sitting and place the hands together in front of the body palms flat against one another with the elbows pointed out.

➢ Press the hands together hard, for as long as possible, or for a designated time period while flexing the chest muscles.

LEVEL 2

❖ **(See Push-ups Section)**

Extras

These exercises work multiple areas of the body, so instead of placing them in categories based on body parts as I did previously, I've included them here under extras.

LEVEL 1

❖ **Jumping Jacks.**

➢ Start position: Standing straight with feet together and arms at the sides.

➢ Jump so that the feet land wider than shoulder width apart while simultaneously bringing the hands up to clap above the head.

➢ Jump back to the starting position and repeat continuously.

❖ **Tip and grip.**

This exercise is for forearms and calves.

➢ Start position: Standing straight with feet close together and arms extended out to the sides.

➢ Jump using the calves, making sure to try and keep the knees straight.

➢ At the same time with each jump, squeeze the hands to make fists.

➢ Continue for a specific time period or number of reps.

LEVEL 2

❖ **Mountain Climbers.**

➢ Start position: Push-up position.

➢ Holding the hands in start position, kick the right leg forward bringing the knee up toward the chest.

➢ Now, kick the right leg back while bringing the left leg forward.

➢ Repeat continuously for specific time period or number of reps.

❖ **Squat Thrust.**

➢ Start Position: Standing straight with arms at sides and feet shoulder width apart.

➢ From the standing position, kick the feet back and drop straight down into a push-up position.

➢ Pop back up to the start position.

➢ Repeat.

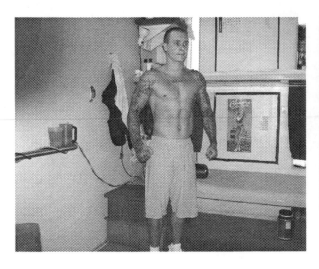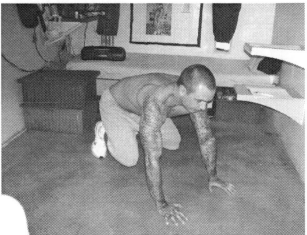

❖ **Burpees (See Push-ups Section)**

My personal favorites.

These are some of my personal favorite exercises along with some of my favorite techniques for performing them. My favorite chest exercises are not listed here, but are listed in the Push-ups section.

Legs

1. **Split Squat.** Using the 1¼ repetition technique.

2. **Step-ups.**

3. **Pick-ups.**

Core Exercises

1. **Hands under sit-up.** Using the top and bottom squeeze technique.

2. **Hanging Knee-up**. Using the negative repetition technique.

3. **Twisting side crunch.** Using the 3-second repetitions technique.

Shoulder Exercises

1.   **Handstand Push-up.**

2.   **Bear crawls.** (Backwards)

3.   **Push-ups.** Using shoulder emphasis techniques (described in Push-up Section)

Back Exercises

1.   **Plyometric Pull-ups.** Using the descending repetitions technique.

2.   **Around the world Pull-**ups. Using the forced repetitions technique.

3.   **Supermans.**

Arm Exercises

1.   **Crab walks.**

2.   **Push-ups.** Using the arms emphasis techniques (described in the Push-ups Section)

3.   **Hanging grips.** Using the descending repetitions technique.

Warm-ups/Cool downs

Although most guys I have seen working out never or rarely use them, warm-ups and cool downs are important to training and should always be included in a workout. Without going into any details or science, here are a few reasons that warm-ups and cool downs are and should be included in workouts.

Warm-ups:

- Increase the physical performance during the workout.

- Help prevent premature fatigue.

- Decrease the likelihood of injury.

- Prepare connective tissue (ligaments and tendons) to handle the stress of exercise.

- Serve as a transition to help the body adjust to new higher level of activity.

Cool downs:

- Serve as a transition to help readjust the body to lower levels of activity.

- Aids in recovery.

When warm-ups are done, they should be progressive, meaning they should gradually get the body warming up. The wrong way to warm-up would be to do too much, too fast, and tire the body out.

Warm-ups can be simply a light jog or some calisthenic exercise.

Here is an example of two warm-ups that I commonly use:

- Light jog for 5-10 minutes. Followed by 5-10 minutes of stretching.

- Calisthenic exercises done in a circuit (in succession). 50 jumping jacks; 50 knee-ups; 50 standing toe touches; 50 squats; 50 push-ups; 50 side bends; 50

shoulder circles. This usually takes me around 6 minutes. Followed by 5-10 minutes of stretching.

Everyone is different so the second warm-up although is a warm-up for me, may be too difficult for some people to perform as a warm-up. It is simply an example. As I perform the calisthenic warm-up the pace starts slow and gradually increases.

For a cool down I will often perform the same things I do for a warm-up. Except for instead of gradually increasing the pace I gradually decrease the pace; stretching precedes the cool down rather than following it.

Jump Training

Jump training, also known as plyometric exercise, utilizes quick, explosive, and jumping type movements to produce explosiveness and power.

Plyometric exercises have long been a part of athletic training and are increasingly being used in all kinds of fitness settings. Plyometrics can be utilized in more than one way depending on the desired result. First, they can be used to improve specific components of fitness such as explosiveness, power endurance, and agility. In addition, they can be used simply to add intensity to a workout, especially when there is little time available for exercise.

These exercises are some of the most stressful on the body. For this reason they are usually not recommended for beginners. Also, because they are a stressful type of exercise, it is important that a thorough and proper warm-up precedes a workout that will include plyometric exercises. The warm-up should include some sets that are a light version of the specific exercise to be performed, say at a quarter-speed up to half-speed. For instance, when squat jumps will be performed as part of the workout, the warm up should include two or three light sets of squat jumps at say 50% of maximal effort.

So as not to turn this into a long discussion about Plyometrics, I will not go into any great detail regarding the science behind, or specific applications of them. For further information including the science and history behind Plyometrics, there are a number of books available. I would personally recommend Donald A. Chu PhD. Dr. Chu is a well-known and respected authority on Plyometrics. One of his books that I have found very useful is *Jumping into Plyometrics*.

The following section provides some samples of plyometric exercises.

Plyometric Exercises

These exercises should be performed quickly and explosively. Do not land hard on any surfaces, but instead land and immediately take off again. All of these exercises are **Level 3** intensity exercises.

❖ **Jump and tuck knees to chest.**

➤ Start Position: Standing straight, with arms at sides and feet shoulder width apart.

➤ Jump straight up as high as possible while bringing the knees to the chest; quickly grab the knees with the hands while in the air, and land in starting position.

➤ Once the feet touch the ground repeat immediately.

❖ **Squat Jump.**

Basically the same as performing a squat, but adding a jump to the upward phase of the exercise.

➤ Start Position: Standing straight, with arms at sides and feet shoulder width apart.

➤ Drop down quickly into the lowered squat position and jump as high as possible straight up.

➤ Land in start position and repeat immediately.

❖ **Jump with heel kick.**

➤ Start Position: Standing straight, with arms at sides and feet shoulder width apart.

> Jump straight up and kick the buttocks with the heels. Do not squat down to jump.

> Land in start position and repeat immediately.

❖ **Pike Jump.**

> Start Position: Standing straight, with arms at sides and feet shoulder width apart.

> Jump straight up and bring the legs straight out in front of the body, while reaching out to touch the toes.

> Land in start position and repeat immediately.

❖ **Lateral Jump.**

> Start Position: Standing straight, with arms at sides and feet shoulder width apart.

> Jump up and to the side to land a few feet to the side from the starting point.

> Once landed, immediately jump back the opposite way. Or an object can be jumped over from side to side.

❖ **Jump over object.**

> Start Position: Standing straight, with arms at sides and feet shoulder width apart in front of the object to be cleared.

> Jump over object by bringing the knees up to clear the object being jumped. (Not by squatting down to jump.)

> Land, turn around, and jump the other way.

❖ **Frog Jumps.**

> Start position: Squatted down completely with the hands touching the ground (like a frog.)

> Leap up and forward as high and as far as possible.

> Land in start position and repeat immediately.

❖ **Diagonal Jumps.**

➤ Start Position: Standing straight, with arms at sides and feet together.

➤ Jump in a diagonal direction from left to right, keeping the feet together. Land and jump from the balls of the feet.

➤ Once landed, repeat the jump in the opposite direction. Repeat jumping diagonally back and forth.

❖ **Forward Jumps.**

➤ Start Position: Standing straight, with arms at the sides and feet shoulder width apart.

➤ Jump forward as far as possible, swinging the arms to gain momentum.

➤ Upon landing repeat immediately.

❖ **Stair Hops.**

➤ Start Position: Standing in front of a set of stairs, with arms at sides (for balance), or hands on back of head, and feet shoulder width apart.

➤ Jump up to the second or third step.

➤ Upon landing, repeat immediately all the way to the top skipping one or two stairs at a time.

❖ **One Leg Zig Zag.**

➤ Start position: Standing on one foot.

➤ Jump diagonally back and forth from left to right, jumping and landing on the same foot.

➤ Upon landing repeat immediately.

❖ **Step-ups.**

➤ Start position: Standing straight, with arms to the sides and feet shoulder width apart in front of step, box, or other elevated object.

➤ Like the step-up exercise previously shown in the singles section, except when stepping up, explode upward starting with the right foot on box and the left foot on the ground, and landing with left foot on box and the right foot on the ground.

➤ Upon landing repeat immediately back and forth.

❖ Jump from box to box.

➤ Start position: Standing on box or other elevated surface and facing another box.

➤ Jump down from the box.

➤ Upon landing on the ground, jump quickly up to the other box.

➤ Turn and repeat in the opposite direction.

❖ Jump up to box.

➤ Start Position: Standing straight, with arms at sides and feet shoulder width apart, and in front of box or other elevated surface.

➤ Jump up to box, and then jump back down to land in start position.

➤ Repeat immediately.

❖ Jump up to. (Push-ups)

➤ Start Position: Push-up position between two boxes.

➤ Explode upward to land with both hands on boxes.

➤ Next, push-up from the boxes to land in the starting position on the floor between the two boxes.

➤ Repeat.

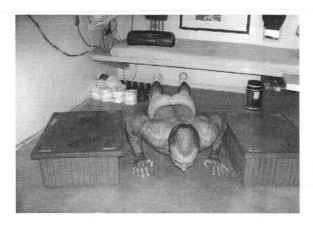
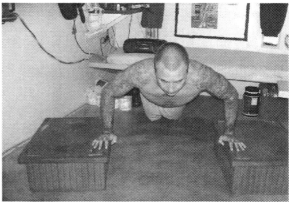

❖ Claps (Push-ups)

➢   Start Position: Push-up position.

➢   Explode upward so that both hands leave the ground.

➢   Clap the hands together.

➢   Land in start position and repeat immediately.

❖ Body Hops. (Push-ups)

➢   Start Position: Push-up position.

➢   Explode upward and jump off of the ground with both hands and both feet.

➢   Land and repeat immediately.

❖ Handstand Jump. (Requires a partner)

➢   Start position: Standing straight up on hands with partner to hold the feet.

➢   Explode upward to jump off of the ground with hands.

➢   Land and repeat immediately.

❖ Switch grip (Pull-ups)

➢   Start position: Hanging on pull-up bar with pronated (overhand) grip, and hands about shoulder width apart.

➢   Explode upward with pull-up motion so that the hands come off of the bar, and while in the air, switch the hands to the chin-up grip (supinated palms facing the body.)

➢   Catch the bar on the way down with the chin-up grip.

➢   Now perform the chin-up explosively and catch the bar in the pull-up position.

➢   Repeat back and forth.

❖ Hop up (Pull-ups)

➢   Start position: Standing straight with arms at sides and feet shoulder width apart in front of a pull-up bar.

➢   Jump up to pull-up bar and perform one pull-up then let go of the bar and drop down.

➢   Land in start position and repeat immediately.

❖   **Quick step-ups. (See Single [Leg] Exercises)**

❖   **Plyometric Pull-ups. (See Single [Back] Exercises)**

My Personal Favorites.

These are some of my favorite plyometric exercises.

1.   **Jump and tuck knees to chest.**
2.   **Jump up to box.**
3.   **Jump up to (push-ups).**
4.   **Switch grip pull-ups.**
5.   **Hop up pull-ups.**
6.   **Plyometric pull-ups.**

667 Push-Ups

One of the simplest but best all around exercises used everywhere from elementary school P.E. classes to special armed forces training is the push-up. I'm sure most people know what a push-up is, and most have probably done a push-up or two in their lifetime. Many may not know however, of how powerful the push-up can be. So why did I include over 600 kinds of push-ups?

First of all, as I have already mentioned, doing exercises in different ways adds variety to your workouts. Doing the same old thing every time gets boring. When your workout is simple and boring, pretty soon you may stop looking forward to doing it. This lack of motivation to workout is counterproductive to improving fitness levels. However, when new exercises and challenges are constantly added to your workouts, it becomes new each time and gives you something to look forward to. When there is an exercise you haven't tried yet, you may find it a little more interesting than doing the same exercises as last time. With push-ups, you can simply do the same old thing, or you can challenge yourself in over six hundred ways. I don't know about you, but I think six hundred is far more interesting than just one or two. Six hundred different ways of performing push-ups is a surefire way to take the routine out of your routine!

Another thing that I have previously mentioned is that challenging your body in different and unique ways can help improve performance levels. If you constantly do the same type of exercise, the same way, for the same number of repetitions, your body will eventually become very efficient at doing that routine. But if you want to improve beyond that point, then you will need to increase the challenge of your workout and push the body further. Having six hundred variations of an exercise can definitely challenge the body in new ways!

Consider also that push-ups are not just an exercise for the chest as is sometimes believed. Push-ups actually challenge most of the body in one way or another. Push-ups can be altered to apply more workload to certain areas of the body, as will be shown in this section. One can place more work on the chest, shoulders, arms, or even the core, by adjusting the way in which the exercise is performed.

In this section there are a number of techniques for performing each repetition that can be applied to each kind of push-up. Combined, the different push-ups, along with the techniques for performing them, provide for well over 667 push-ups. I just liked calling it 667 ways to do push-ups.

I realize that over 600 kinds of push-ups may seem excessive, and even ridiculous to some people. However, I like having a large arsenal of exercises at my disposal. Some people may feel as though they don't need that many. Perhaps then if they found ten out of the six hundred that they liked, that would be ten that they didn't have before. For those that I have trained, my suggestion was to try three or four kinds at every workout in which push-ups would be performed, starting with the ones that look most interesting on paper. All of those guys found some push-ups that they really liked and continue to use them still.

While I have been writing this book people have been hearing rumors that I have come up with "a million ways to do push-ups", and they are some times skeptical. Once I show them a push-up or two, the guys who thought they would be able to handle any kind of push-up are amazed when they can't even complete five! Some people may be thinking, "I can do 100 push-ups no problem, what do I need all these different kinds for?" Those people are the perfect candidate to try something new, as obviously they've already mastered the regular push-up.

Techniques for Performing Each Repetition

Like the techniques that I listed in the single exercises section, these techniques can also be applied to the push-up exercises in this book. These techniques are used to add variety, to add new dimensions to the exercise, and to increase the ways in which the muscles are trained.

Example #1 Rather than simply performing the stagger push-up as normal, the stagger push-up is performed using the lower-body elevated technique so that the feet are placed on a raised surface.

Example #2 Instead of performing the Up and over box push-up as normal, the push-up is performed using the 3-second repetition technique.

1.   Jump.

The jump is performed by jumping completely off of the ground with the hands on the concentric (upward) phase of the push-up. This can be made a little more challenging by clapping the hands together before landing back on the ground.

Why? This technique helps to improve power and explosiveness.

2.   Negative Reps.

Negative repetitions are performed by slowly lowering the body toward the ground during the eccentric (downward) phase of the push-up. The body may be lowered from 3 seconds to as long as one wishes. The concentric (upward) phase is performed at normal speed.

Why? This technique increases the time in which the muscles are placed under tension and therefore increases the workload of a given set. It can help to increase muscular endurance as well.

3.   3 Second Reps.

3-second repetitions are performed slowly on the upward and downward phases of the push-up. They are basically slow motion push-ups performed at 3 seconds down and 3 seconds up.

Why? This technique increases the time in which the muscles are placed under tension and therefore increases the workload of a given set. It can help to improve muscular endurance as well.

4.   Top and Bottom Pause.

Using the top and bottom pause, the body is held and all muscles are flexed for a period of one full second or more at the very top and the very bottom of the push-up. These can also be done as top, middle, and bottom pauses. Rather than pausing to flex only at the top and bottom of the push-up, also pause at the halfway point.

Why? This technique adds a brief isometric contraction at the top and bottom of the range of motion, which helps to increase the workload.

5.   1¼ Reps.

One of my favorites, one-and-a-quarter repetitions are performed by lowering the body completely during the eccentric (downward) phase, and then coming up only about a quarter of the way, before lowering again to the bottom and then all the way to the top. So, one performs a quarter of a push-up, followed by a full push-up.

Why? Performing 1¼ repetitions, (say ten reps), you not only get ten full repetitions, you also get ten quarter-repetitions that add strength and endurance to that specific shortened range of motion. This also increases the workload by increasing the amount of time that the muscles are placed under tension.

6. 1,2,3's.

1,2,3's are a variation of the 1¼ reps. The difference being that the first repetition comes up off of the ground only a couple of inches, the second repetition comes up even further to two-thirds of the way up, and the third repetition is a full range rep or all of the way to the top.

Why? Performing 1,2,3's, you get the same added benefit of the 1¼ reps, but with even more added workload per repetition.

7. Upper-body elevated.

Upper body elevated push-ups are simply those that are performed at an angle of decline. This is done simply by placing the hands on an elevated object or surface.

Why? This adds a new angle to the push-up and takes some of the resistance off of the exercise, making it easier to perform.

8. Lower-body elevated.

Lower-body elevated is exactly the opposite of the upper-body elevated push-ups. Instead of placing the hands on an elevated surface, the feet are placed on an elevated surface.

Why? This adds a new angle to the exercises and adds resistance to the upper body, making it more difficult to perform.

9. Fingertips.

Rather than performing the push-up on the palms of the hands, the push-ups are done on the fingertips.

Why? Fingertip push-ups can really strengthen the hands and add a lot of difficulty to the exercise.

10. Knuckles.

Rather than performing the push-ups on the palms of the hands, the push-ups are done on the knuckles.

Why? Knuckle push-ups are used by martial artists to toughen the hands, and they keep the wrist straight rather than bent as they are when performing a push-up on the palms of the hands. This creates a whole new angle for the wrists. (Good for improving punching power by strengthening the wrists in that straightened angle).

11. Knee up.

The knee up is done by performing a push-up and when at the top position, flexing at the hip to raise the knee toward the chest, one knee at a time. Basically, one lifts a knee between each repetition.

Why? The knee-up creates a new element to the push-up exercise. It adds a hip flexor movement and adds work to the core.

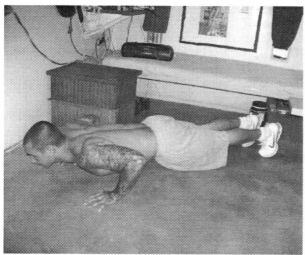 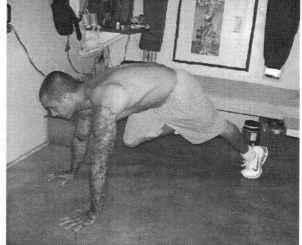

12. One leg up.

This technique is performed by starting in the push-up position. Then, raising one leg up high behind the body and holding it there until the set is complete.

Why? One leg up technique adds a new element to the push-up. It increases the isometric resistance of the lower back and buttocks and adds to the difficulty of core stabilization of the push-up.

13. Feet wide apart.

Normally when performing the push-up the feet are placed together. Using this technique, the feet are placed from several inches apart, to as wide as one may get them apart.

Why? Placing the feet wide apart creates a different base of support and therefore changes the core stabilization of the exercise.

14.   Ascending Reps.

Using this technique, one does a number of push-ups, stands up, and then does a set of one more push-up than before. Example: Do three push-ups, stand, do four push-ups, stand, do five push-ups etc.

Why? Ascending repetitions are a good way to help to push the body farther than it is accustomed to.

15.   Descending Reps.

Descending repetitions are just the opposite of the ascending repetitions. The technique is performed by doing a certain number of reps, standing, and then dropping to do a set of one less rep than before. Example: do ten push-ups, stand, do nine push-ups, stand, do eight push-ups, etc.

Why? Descending repetitions help to push the body farther than it is accustomed to, and are easier than ascending repetitions because you are doing one less than before as opposed to one more than before.

16.   Short Burns.

A popular method, short burns are repetitions that only come a few inches from the ground on the concentric (upward) phase of the push-up, and are done at a high rate of speed. They can be done anywhere within the full range of motion.

Why? Short burns apply all of the workload to a specific range within the full range of motion and keep the muscles under constant tension.

17.   Burpees.

Burpees are a great way to add intensity and a cardio element to push-ups. To perform burpees start by standing up straight then, drop down from the standing position to the push-up position. Next, perform a push-up, then, hop back up to the standing position.

Why? Burpees change the push-up to a whole body exercise and add cardio work to the exercise.

18.   Elevators.

Elevators are performed by starting at the top of the push-up position and lowering to the bottom of the full range of motion. From the bottom, short push-ups are done to slowly raise the body back to the top of the push-up position. It should take around twenty short pushes to get to the top (1 rep), and should be done at a pace that takes around twenty seconds for each rep.

Why? Elevators add workload to the push-up by increasing the time that the muscles are placed under tension.

The Push-ups.

Following are over 50 different ways in which to perform the push-ups themselves. The techniques listed previously are applied to each different kind of push-up to create hundreds of different ways to do push-ups. Note: not all techniques can be applied to every push-up.

There are also categories of intensity Levels 1-3, as with all of the exercises in this book. Level 1 being the easiest, Level 3 the hardest to perform.

LEVEL 1

❖ Shoulder width.

➢ Shoulder width push-ups are the normal push-up. Both hands are positioned beneath, but slightly wider than the shoulders with the fingers pointed forward and the feet are placed together.

❖ Hands wide.

➢ As the name implies, rather than positioning the hands slightly wider than shoulder width, the hands are placed much wider with the fingers still pointed forward.

❖ Hands narrow.

➢ The opposite of the Hands wide push-up, for this type of push-up, the hands are positioned very close together with the fingers pointed forward and the elbows tucked in close to the body.

❖ **Hands pointed out.**

➤ Hands pointed out push-ups are performed by placing the hands in any wide or narrow position, but turning the hands so that instead of pointing forward, they point out to each side.

LEVEL 2

❖ **Diamonds.**

➤ Diamond push-ups are great for putting a greater workload on the triceps muscles. Diamonds are done by positioning the hands directly beneath the middle of the chest and making a diamond shape with the hands by touching the thumbs and index fingers together. Elbows are held close in to the body.

❖ **Staggered.**

➤ Staggered push-ups are performed by placing one hand in the shoulder width position, while positioning the other hand a few inches forward from the body.

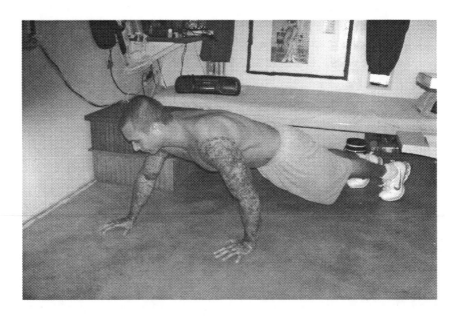

❖ **Hands pointed in.**

➤ Hands pointed in are simply the opposite of hands pointed out push-ups. The hands are placed in any wide or narrow position and then turned to point inward so that the fingers from both hands are pointed at each other. Keep the elbows out away from the body.

❖ **One in One out.**

➤ One in one out pushups are performed by positioning one hand shoulder width with the elbow tucked in close to the body, while the other hand is placed as wide as possible. Both hands are still pointed forward.

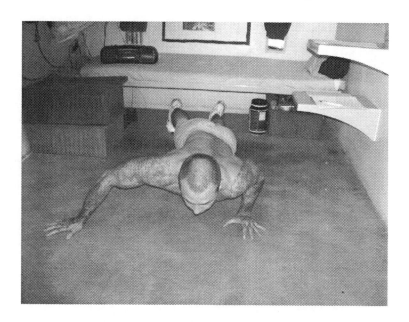

❖ **One hand on ball.**

➤ One hand on ball push-ups are performed by placing one hand on the ground, and one hand on a medicine ball or some other raised surface. This push-up is similar to the one hand on wall push-up in the level 3 section. The difference between the two kinds of push-ups is that with one hand on ball push-ups, both hands contribute to the exercise, whereas with one hand on the wall, the hand that is on the wall cannot be used to help lift the body, and they are much harder.

❖ **Raise one hand.**

➤ Raise one hand push-ups are performed by completing a push-up, and then raising one's hand in the air, by twisting the torso to point the hand at the sky. This makes the body into a T shape. This is repeated so that first the right hand is raised, and then the left hand is raised.

❖ Up and over.

➢ Start in the push-up position, and to the side of an elevated object such as a box or a medicine ball etc. Perform one push-up on the side of the box. Then, going from right to left, put the left hand on the box and perform another push-up. Next, the right hand is placed on the box and another push-up is performed. Followed by the left hand being placed on the ground and another push-up. Finally, the right hand is placed on the ground for a fifth push-up. Then repeat in the opposite direction.

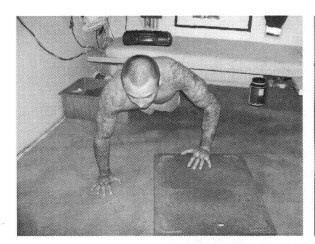 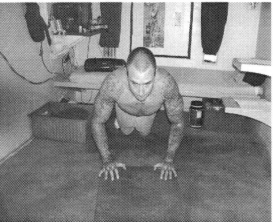

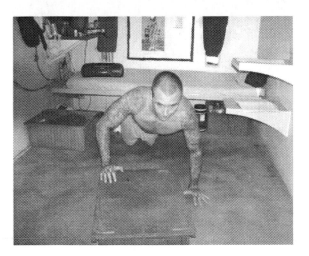

❖ Dive into.

➢ Start in the shoulder width push-up position. Then, instead of pushing straight up and down, dive into the push-up as is shown in the photos.

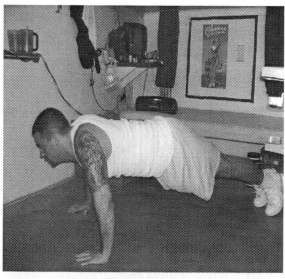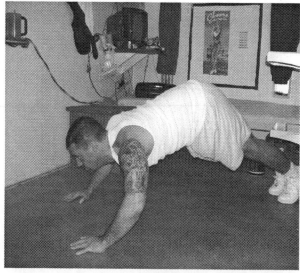

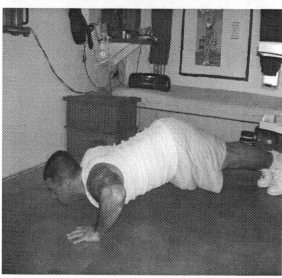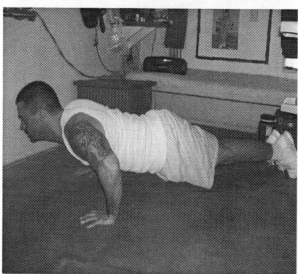

❖ **Deck of cards.**

➢ These push-ups are performed using a deck of playing (poker) cards. The deck of cards is placed on the ground, and face down. The person performing the push-ups then positions himself, in push-up position, next to the deck of cards. He then turns over one card and does the number of push-ups that are on that card. If he turns over the five of clubs he will do five etc. The value for Jacks is 11; Queens, 12; Kings, 13. He continues until the entire deck has been flipped over one card at a time. These can also be done by flipping a card, doing the designated number of push-ups, and then standing for a few seconds between each card. The total number of push-ups from an entire deck of cards is 364.

❖ **Bear crawl.**

➤ Most any of the push-ups can be performed with the bear crawl although usually the regular shoulder width push-up is used. Perform this push-up by getting into bear crawl position and taking two to four steps forward with the hands, as with the bear crawl exercise described earlier. Then, complete any number of reps (usually one or two is best) and continue crawling and stopping to do push-ups every couple of steps. It's more challenging than it sounds.

❖ **Backward bear crawl.**

➤ This push-up is the same as the bear crawl except the bear crawl is done backwards. The backwards bear crawl is far more challenging than the forward version.

❖ **Drag foot bear crawl.**

➤ Again, this exercise is performed the same as the bear crawl push-up, except that only the hands are used to crawl, and the feet are dragged to add difficulty to the exercise.

❖ **Stagger crawl.**

➤ These push-ups are performed by starting in the staggered push-up position, performing a staggered push-up, taking one step forward or backward with the hands into the opposite staggered position, and performing another staggered push-up.

❖ **Sideway crawl.**

➤ This is another version of the bear crawl with the difference being instead of crawling forward or backward, the person performing the exercise crawls sideways. First, one or two push-ups are performed, then one or two steps sideways is taken with the hands and feet, followed by one or two more push-ups and so on.

❖ **Wall crawl two handed.**

➤ This exercise can definitely be felt in the shoulders. The wall crawl is performed by starting in shoulder width push-up position next to a wall, with the head closest to the wall and the feet furthest from the wall. Going from left to right, the right hand is placed on the wall with the palm flat against the wall, followed by the left hand. Taking one step at a time, with the right hand followed by the left hand, four steps are taken along the wall. Then the right and left hands are placed on the ground and a push-up is performed. This is then repeated in the opposite direction, back and forth from left to right and right to left. So, the hands are used to hold the body up and crawl along a wall. Another option is complete the entire length of say a gym wall in one direction and then back again.

❖ Tag Team. (Requires a Partner)

➢ This push-up is done with a partner. It is performed with the two partners facing each other in push-up position, each performs a push-up at the same time, and at the top position of the push-up both take their right hand and reach out to tag the other partners hand. This is followed by another push-up and a left hand tag.

❖ Tag Team crawl to middle. (Requires a Partner)

➢ This exercise is a combination of the tag team and bear crawl push-ups. The two partners begin a few feet apart, in the push-up position and facing each other. They then bear crawl toward one another, perform a push-up, and then tag each other. They then bear crawl backward to the start position and repeat.

❖ Wheelbarrow. (Requires a Partner)

➢ This is another push-up that requires a partner. This exercise is performed by having partner A in push-up position, and partner B standing behind his or her feet. Partner B then grabs partner A's feet and brings them up to waist level. Partner A performs a push-up and then crawls forward with partner B holding his feet (like a wheelbarrow.) He continues to crawl forward and or backward performing a push-up every few steps.

❖ 3 to 300. (Requires a Partner)

➢ This exercise requires one or more partners. This example uses 3 partners. With three partners each in push-up position the first performs a push-up and calls out "one". The next partner then performs a push-up and calls out "two". The third then follows and calls out "three". Back to the first partner who does his push-up and calls out "four". This is repeated until 300 push-ups (or any chosen number of push-ups) are completed. All of the partners must remain in the push-up position until the set is complete.

❖ **3 to the middle. (Requires a Partner)**

➢ This one is a combination of the tag team to the middle and 3 to 300 push-ups. To perform this exercise, three or more partners all start facing each other in the push-up position, and encircling a common point that is in the middle of all of the partners. The first partner then bear crawls to the middle point, does a push-up and calls out "one". He then waits in the middle for the second partner to crawl to the middle, and tag his hand at which point he crawls back to his starting point. The second partner then performs his push-up and calls out "two". He then waits for the third partner to tag him, and so on until the set is completed by reaching a chosen number of push-ups. As with the 3 to 300 push-ups, all partners must remain in the push-up position until the set is completed.

❖ **Pike between.**

➢ This push-up and the next five push-ups are simple, and just add an exercise to be performed between each repetition of push-ups. As is already obvious, any exercise can be done in between each rep. I have included six that I like. This push-up is simply done by performing a push-up, and then performing a pike at the hips (which is; leaving the hands on the ground, and jumping forward with the feet, and then kicking the feet back to the start position) and then repeating. See photos.

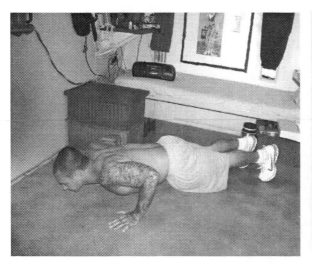 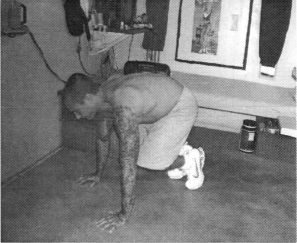

❖ **Somersault between.**

➢ Simply perform a push-up, then somersault forward and perform another push-up and repeat. This can be done in one direction or can be done by somersaulting forward and then backward.

❖ **Mt. Climber between.**

➢ Perform a push-up and perform one repetition of Mountain climber with both feet. Repeat.

❖ **Sit through between.**

➢ This push-up is performed by completing a push-up followed by a sit through. Then, pop back into push-up position, perform another push-up, followed by a sit through in the opposite direction. It is repeated back and forth. These ones are pretty challenging. See photos for the sit through exercise.

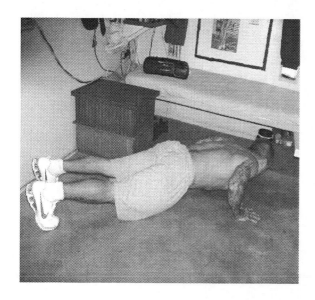 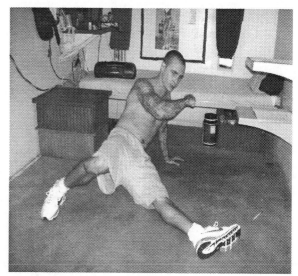

❖ **Plank between.**

➢ Perform one to ten push-ups, and then plank for ten seconds, and then repeat.

❖ **Bird dog between.**

➢   Perform one to ten push-ups, then bird dog for ten seconds and then repeat.

5 Burpee samples

❖ **Burpee #1.**

This is the simplest burpee.

➢   Start position: standing straight with arms at the sides.

➢   Next, drop down to the push-up position.

➢   Then perform a push-up.

➢   Finally, pop back up to standing position and repeat.

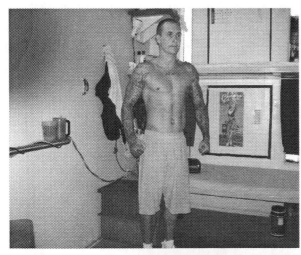 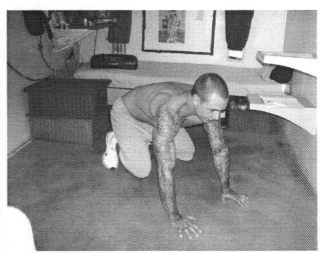

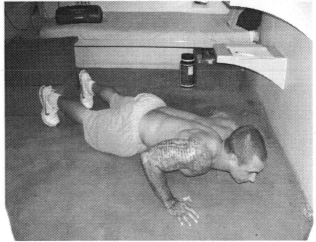

❖ Burpee #2.

This one is my favorite burpee. This burpee is performed similar to the first burpee except for an added exercise.

➢ Start position: Standing upright with the hands at the sides.

➢ Next, drop down into push-up position.

➢ Then, perform a push-up, followed by a sit through.

➢ Finally, pop back into standing position and repeat.

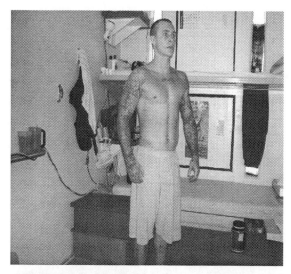
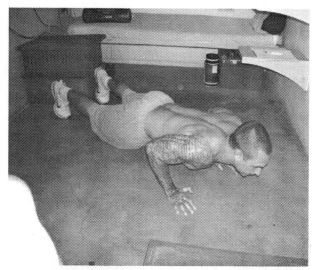
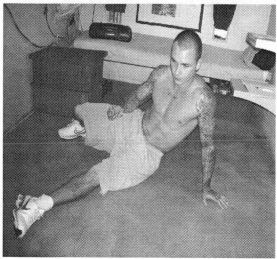
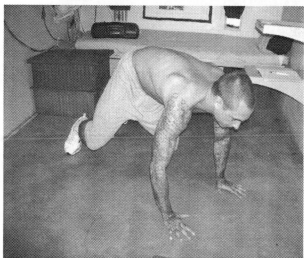

❖ Burpee #3.

This burpee simply adds the Pike motion instead of the sit through.

➢   Start position: Standing upright hands at the sides.

➢   Next, drop down to push-up position.

➢   Then, perform a push-up, followed by the Pike.

➢   Finally, pop back up to standing position.

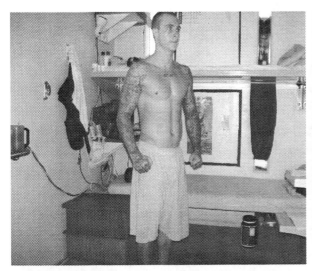
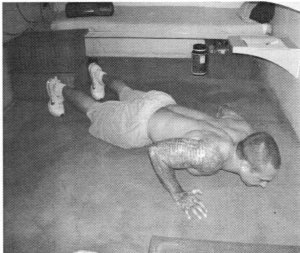
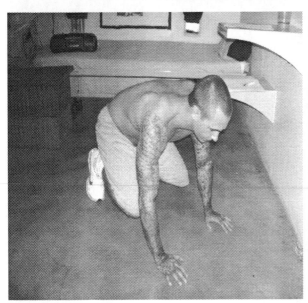
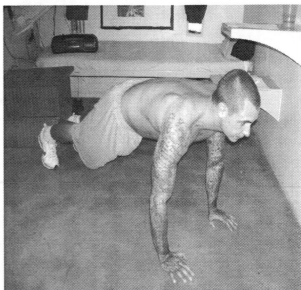

❖ Burpee #4.

Another version of the regular burpee that simply adds a movement.

➤ Start in standing position.

➤ Next, drop down to push-up position and perform a push-up.

➤ Then, pop back up to standing position, and as soon as the feet hit the ground, jump straight up as high as possible.

➤ Repeat.

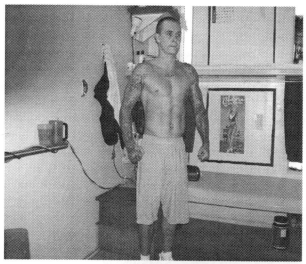
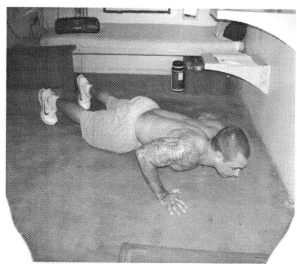
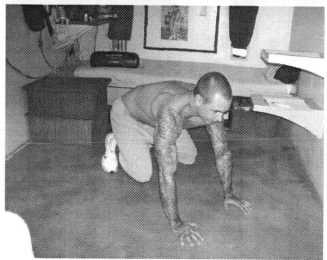

❖ Burpee #5.

There's a little more to this one.

➤ Start in standing position.

➤ Next, raise both hands (made into fists) high above the head.

➤ Then, in one motion, hit the torso with the fists, squat down to the bottom of the squat position, and drop down into push-up position.

➤ Then, perform a push-up, and bring the left knee up, followed by a push-up with the right knee brought up.

➤ Finally, pop back up to standing position and bring the left knee up, and then the right knee up.

➤ Repeat.

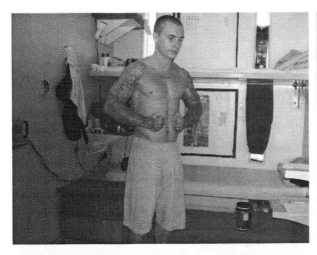 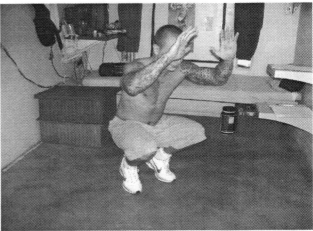

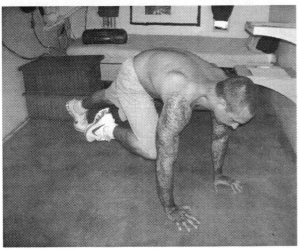 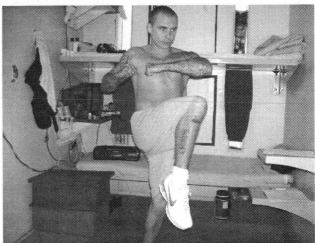

LEVEL 3

❖ **North South.**

➤ North south push-ups are performed by placing one hand as far forward from the body as one can reach with the fingers pointed forward, while the other hand is placed as far in the other direction as one can reach, with the fingers pointed toward the feet.

❖ **One-handed.**

➤ One-handed push-ups are another of my favorites. These push-ups will make a person soar in all kinds of places. They are usually performed with the feet wide and one hand shoulder width with the other hand tucked behind the back.

❖ **One and a half.**

➤ This is a great one for those who are not quite strong enough to perform one-handed push-ups. The one and a half push-up is performed by placing one hand shoulder width with the elbow held close to the body with the other hand extended as far out to the side as possible and only the fingertips touch the ground. The hand that is extended out is only used to balance the body and assist the hand that is doing most of the work (the one next to the body.) The reason for the name of course is because this push-up is almost, but not quite, a one-handed push-up.

❖ **One-hand/Two-hand.**

➤ The one-hand two-hand is simply alternating from a one-handed push-up to a two-handed push-up. The one-hand two-hand is when first, a one-handed push-up is performed. The other hand is then placed on the ground, and a two-handed push-up is performed. This is repeated back and forth.

❖ **One-hand/1½.**

➤ As in the one-hand two-hand push-up, the one-hand 1½ is simply alternating between a one-handed push-up and a one and a half push-up. First, a one handed push-up is performed. Then, the other hand is placed on the ground in the one and a half push-up position, and a one and a half push-up is performed. This is repeated back and forth.

❖ **Two-hand/1 ½.**

➤ Again, this is simply alternating between a two-handed push-up and a one and a half push-up. First, the two-handed pushup is performed. Then, the hands are placed in the one and a half push-up position, and a one and a half push-up is performed. This is repeated back and forth.

❖ **One-handed alternating.**

➤ The one-handed alternating is the way I prefer to do my one-handed push-ups. By alternating back and forth from the left hand to the right hand, I complete more total repetitions. These push-ups are performed by first competing a one-handed push-up with the left hand, and then switching to the right hand and performing a one-handed push-up. This is repeated back and forth.

❖ **One hand on wall.**

➤ The one hand on wall push-up is performed by positioning one's self with the head close to a wall (with the feet furthest from the wall). One hand is then placed on the ground and the other is placed with the palm flat against the wall. These are actually pretty challenging, and are similar to one-handed push-ups.

❖ **Divers.**

➤ Divers are one of the hardest push-ups that I know of, at least for me anyway. They are performed by placing the hands as far out in front of the body as possible (as if diving into a swimming pool) with the palms on the floor and hands together. The body is then raised up by pushing with the hands against the floor. This one takes a lot of shoulder and core strength.

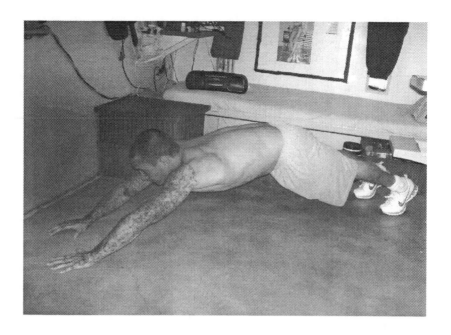

❖ **Knife fighters.**

➢ Knife fighters are another tough one. These are performed by placing the hands far out in front of the body like with the diver push-up. Except that instead of the palms being placed flat on the ground, a fist is made with both hands and the hands are then placed pinky side down on the ground. (Like stabbing a knife into the ground). The proper way to perform this push-up is to lift with the chest and core muscles (not bending at the elbow). Otherwise this exercise will simply turn into a triceps extension.

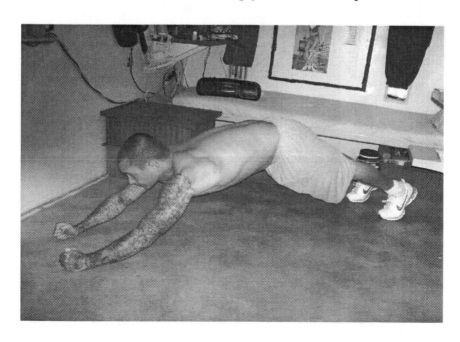

❖ **Knife fighter/staggered.**

➢ This push-up is the same as the knife fighter, except that one hand is placed further out in front of the body than the other hand like with the stagger push-up. Again, the proper way to lift the body is with the chest and core muscles (not bending at the elbow).

❖ **Knife fighter 1½'s.**

➢ This push-up is performed by placing one hand in the knife fighter position, while the other hand is placed in the one and a half position (out to the side and on fingertips.) The workload then, is placed on the knife fighter side.

❖ **'Round the clock.**

➢ These are performed by starting in the shoulder width push-up position. From here, the right hand is moved forward from the body as if pointed toward the 12 on a clock. Then, a push-up is performed with the hands in this new position. On the upward motion of the next pushup the right hand is moved to the position where the 1 would be on the clock. This is repeated until the right hand gets to the position of the 6 on a clock, (next to the hip with the fingers pointed toward the feet). The next repetition begins with the right hand in the shoulder width position and the left hand placed in the 6 position. The push-ups continue with the left hand moving from 6 to 7,8, and 9 etc. Once the left hand reaches the 12 position, repeat the set in reverse. This makes a set of 24.

❖ **Wall crawl one handed.**

➢ This exercise is a combination of the wall crawl and the one hand on wall push-ups. A wall crawl in one direction is followed by placing one hand on the ground, leaving the other hand on the wall, and performing a one hand on wall push-up. Then, wall crawl back the other direction and so on. (It is the same as the wall crawl push-up except that only one hand comes off of the wall to do each push-up.

All Plyometrics

❖ **(See the Jump Training section for 3 more push-ups)**

❖ **Side to Side.**

➢ Start in push-up position.

➢ Drop down quickly and explode upward, jumping with both hands to the left.

➢ Upon landing, quickly drop down and explode upward, jumping back to the right.

➢ Repeat back and forth.

❖ **Stagger switch.**

➢ Start in the staggered push-up position.

➢ Drop down quickly and explode upward, jumping off the ground with the hands, and switch the hand positions.

➢ Repeat immediately upon landing back and forth.

➢ Clap the hands together during the switch to add difficulty.

❖ **North South switch.**

This one is similar to the stagger switch but much, much harder.

➢ Start in the North South push-up position.

➢ Drop down quickly and explode upward jumping completely off of the ground with both hands and switch hand positions.

➢ Repeat immediately upon landing back and forth.

➢ Clap during the switch to add difficulty.

❖ **1, 2, jump.**

This push-up is like the 1,2,3 repetition technique except the third upward motion is a complete jump off of the ground with the hands.

- ➢ Start in the push-up position.
- ➢ Using the 1,2,3 technique described earlier, the first push-up comes up only a couple of inches off of the ground.
- ➢ The second push-up comes up two thirds of a full rep.
- ➢ Finally, jump completely off of the ground for the third push-up.

❖ Frog hop to clap push-up.

This push-up is brutal, and one of my favorites. It is simply a combination of the frog hop and clap push-up exercises described in the Jump Training section.

- ➢ Start crouched down in the frog hop position.
- ➢ Then, jump up and forward as far as possible.
- ➢ Upon landing drop down quickly to the push-up position and explode off of the ground with a clap push-up.
- ➢ Then, as soon as the hands land back on the ground, quickly kick the feet back into the start position and repeat.

The hands and feet should spend a minimal time in contact with the ground on this one. It does get hard fast.

❖ 1 and 1.

- ➢ This one is simple. Perform one push-up, and then perform any plyometric push-up and repeat back and forth.

❖ Gorillas.

- ➢ Gorillas are performed by starting in the lower-body elevated push-up position, (feet up on a raised surface), and on the knuckles.
- ➢ From the start position, perform an explosive push-up off of the ground.
- ➢ Once the hands leave the ground, beat once on the chest (like a gorilla).
- ➢ Then, land back on the knuckles and repeat immediately.
- ➢ (I always wear gloves when performing these push-ups to protect my knuckles.)

Techniques to change workload emphasis.

These techniques are used to add emphasis or workload to the specific areas of the body. These are just some techniques and not all that are possible.

Chest

These techniques are used to add emphasis to the chest.

1. Elbows are pointed outward and away from the body.

2. The 1¼ repetition technique on the bottom ¼ of the push-up is used.

3. The Short Burn technique at the bottom of the push-up is used.

4. The top and bottom squeeze technique flexing the chest for a full two seconds at the top and bottom is used.

5. The lower body elevated technique is used. This technique is used in conjunction with the hands wide or any of the first four techniques listed above as well.

6. The Diamond push-up, but with the elbows pointed outward is used.

Shoulders

These techniques are used to add more workload to the shoulders.

1. Like the chest technique, elbows pointed outward and away from the body will place more emphasis on the front delts (shoulders).

2. Different crawls push-ups are used. Bear crawls push-ups, and especially the backward version, work the shoulders the best.

3. The wheelbarrow push-up.

4. The Mt. Climber between push-ups is used.

5. The divers push-up is a killer. This will work the muscles that stabilize the shoulder joint more than the delts (shoulder caps) themselves.

6. The knife fighter push-ups are used. Again, this push-up will work the muscles that stabilize the shoulder joint.

7. The 'Round the clock push-ups and the North South push-ups both really work the muscles that stabilize the shoulder joint.

Arms

To place more emphasis and workload to the arms, these techniques are used.

1.   The elbows are tucked in close to the body.

2.   The staggered push-up is used.

3.   The Diamonds push-up is used.

4.   The different Crawls push-ups are used.

5.   The One in one out push-up is used.

6.   The One and a half push-up is used.

7.   The One-handed push-up is used.

Core

To place more emphasis and workload on the core, these techniques are used.

1.   The One leg up technique is used.

2.   The knee-up technique is used.

3.   The divers push-up is used.

4.   The knife fighter push-up is used.

5.   The one-handed push-up is used.

6.   The sit through between push-ups is used.

7.   The plank between push-ups is used.

8.   The birddog between push-up is used.

9.   The pike between push-ups is used.

My 10 personal favorites.

1.   Stagger Push-up and especially the stagger switch.

2.   One handed alternating push-up.

3.   Divers Push-up. Using the fingertip technique.

4.   Bear Crawl Push-up. Using the jump technique for every push-up.

5.   One-handed clap push-up.

6.   Sit through between Push-up.

7.   Diamonds Push-up. Using the 1,2,3 technique.

8.   Gorillas.

9.   Frog hop to clap Push-up.

10.   Pike between push-up. Using the 1¼ technique.

The Most Challenging Push-ups.

These are the push-ups that I, and the people I have trained or worked out with have found to be some of the most difficult.

1.   One-handed push-up. But especially the jump technique, and negative repetition/ fingertip techniques.

2.   Knife fighters. Using the jump technique.

3.   Divers Push-up using any technique.

4.   North South Switch Push-up.

5.   Frog hop to clap Push-up.

Tumbling Drills

So far, bodyweight exercises that improve general fitness levels have been the focus. This section will show some examples of solo and partnered "tumbling drills". These drills are used not only to improve fitness levels, but certain movements and skills related to "tumbling".

There are different reasons that these types of exercises are used. Primarily, they are used to improve the skill and conditioning that are required in combative situations. They are also used to add fun and variety to regular workouts, and to help improve components of fitness such as coordination and agility etc.

In most prisons, this type of training is prohibited. Therefore, training with partners is done covertly. However, the solo drills are often allowed, or go unnoticed looking more like a funky calisthenic exercise. The solo drills are great when there are no partners available to work out with. They are like shadow boxing, and are done with an imaginary opponent.

❖ Shoot/push-up/bear crawl/sit through. (Offense)

➢ Start in crouched standing position.

➢ Shoot forward to push-up potion and perform push-up.

➢ Bear crawl forward two steps and perform sit through.

➢ Stand and repeat.

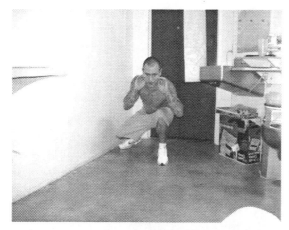
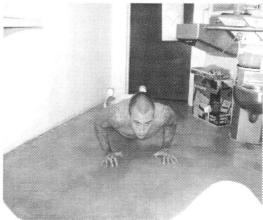
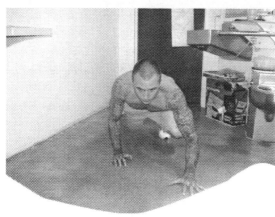
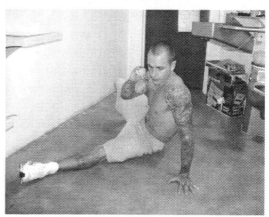

❖ Sprawl/push-up/backward crawl/push-up. (Defense)

➢ Start in crouched standing position.

➢ Sprawl down to push-up position, and perform a push-up.

➢ Bear crawl backward two steps and push-up again.

➢ Stand and repeat.

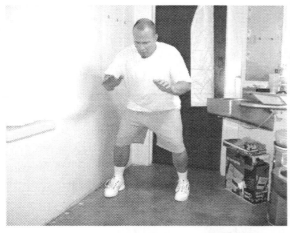 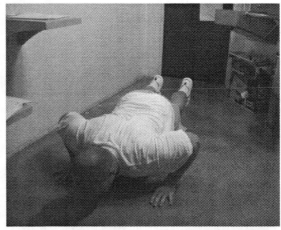

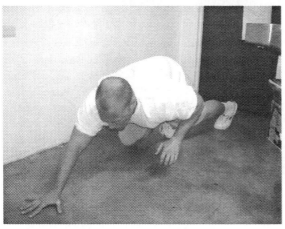 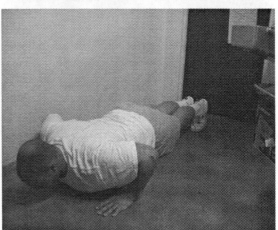

❖ **Shoot/push-up/sit through.**

➢ Start in crouched standing position.

➢ Shoot into push-up position and perform a push-up.

➢ Perform a sit through.

➢ Stand and repeat.

❖ **Sprawl/switch-hand push-up/forward roll.**

➢ Start in crouched standing position.

➢ Sprawl into push-up position, and perform a stagger switch push-up.

➢ Somersault forward, and use the momentum of the somersault to pop back up to feet.

➢ Repeat.

❖ Bear crawl/sit through/ crab walk/hip heist.

➤ Start in bear crawl position.

➤ Bear crawl forward five or six feet, and sit through to the crab walk position (now facing the opposite direction).

➤ Crab walk back to the starting point and hip heist into bear crawl position.

➤ Repeat.

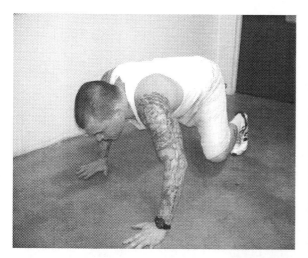
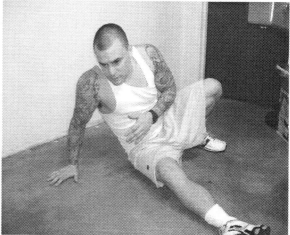
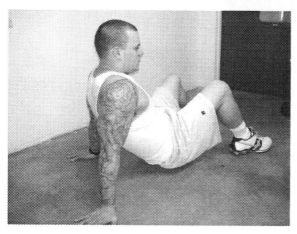
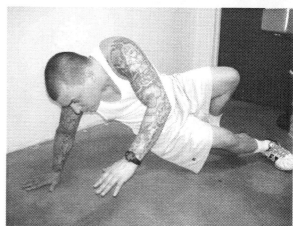

❖ Shoot/push-up/spin/push-up.

➤ Start in crouched standing position.

➤ Shoot forward to push-up position, and perform a push-up.

➤ Without getting up, leave the left hand on the ground and use it as a pivot point to spin around 180 degrees and perform another push-up.

➤ Stand and repeat.

❖ **Frog hop/sprawl/plyo push-up/sit through.**

➢ Start in frog hop position.

➢ Frog hop forward and as high as possible.

➢ As soon as the feet touch the ground upon landing, sprawl into push-up position and perform a push-up with a clap.

➢ Immediately perform a sit through, and then pop back up to frog hop position.

➢ Repeat.

Bag Work

(These drills require a punching bag. When one is not available, inmates will use a mattress that is rolled up and tied with a sheet.)

❖ **Heavy bag/push-ups.**

➢ Start by striking the bag for a designated time, or number of strikes.

➢ When the time, or number of strikes is reached, drop down immediately and perform a number of push-ups.

➢ Repeat. (An example is to start off by hitting the bag for 15 seconds, then drop down and do ten push-ups. Immediately pop back up for 15 more seconds of striking and so on, for 3 minutes.)

❖ **Heavy bag /jumps.**

This is the same as striking the bag with push-ups but with jumps instead. These are much harder.

➢ Strike the bag for designated time period or number of strikes.

➢ Jump, tucking the knees to the chest.

➢ Repeat.

❖ **Heavy bag/sprawl/sit through.**

Again, the bag work is simply alternated with other exercises in this case the sprawl and sit through.

➤   Strike the bag for designated time period or number of reps.

➤   Sprawl and sit through, then pop up to the feet.

➤   Repeat.

❖   **Heavy bag/shoot under/bear crawl/duck walk.**

This one is a little different.

➤   Start by striking the bag for certain time, or number of reps.

➤   If the bag is not already moving because of the strikes, shove it forward.

➤   When the bag comes back toward you, shoot underneath it into bear crawl position.

➤   Bear crawl forward a few feet, then hop up to duck walk position, and duck walk back to the bag.

➤   Repeat.

❖   **Heavy bag 100's.**

Heavy bag 100's are simply striking the bag for a set of 100 strikes. Examples are 100 left hooks, 100 right elbows, or 100 right front kicks etc. They can also be sets of combinations for a hundred reps. Left straight, right hook, left elbow 100 times, for example.

Partnered

(The following drills require at least one partner.)

❖   **Heavy bag/drive.**

Start with partner A holding the bag, and partner B performing the exercise.

➤   Partner B begins by striking the bag as hard and fast as possible with the same kind of strike (all hooks, or all straights etc.)

➤   After a designated time period, or number of strikes, partner B then drives partner A for a certain distance or time. Example: Partner B strikes bag for 30 seconds, he then drives partner A forward for 10 feet. Both partners quickly return to the start, and repeat for 3 minutes.

❖ Heavy bag/defend.

Start with partner A striking the bag, and partner B standing within a couple of feet, and to the side of partner A.

➢ Partner A begins striking the bag with random attacks and combinations, while moving around the bag.

➢ At random intervals, partner B will attempt to shoot on partner A's legs and partner A must defend himself from being taken down. This is repeated for 3-minute rounds.

❖ Drive/push-up.

Start with partners A and B standing face to face.

➢ Partner A drops down and performs a push-up.

➢ After performing the push-up, he drives into partner B and drives partner B for 5 to 10 feet and drops down to perform another push-up.

➢ This is repeated driving forward and stopping every few feet to push-up.

❖ Pick-up/push-up.

Start with partner A standing directly behind partner B.

➢ Partner A squats down grabbing partner B around the waist and lifts partner B up off of the ground, using his legs to lift.

➢ Partner A then takes four steps forward carrying partner B.

➢ Partner A then sets down partner B, and drops down to perform a push-up.

➢ Partner A gets back up and repeats.

❖ Take down/defend.

This is an exercise game or drill. Often times, a score is kept to see who did better. Two partners start by facing one another standing a couple of feet apart. The drill is done in timed rounds such as 3 minutes. Each partner will have a chance at offense and defense.

➢ Partner A starts round 1 as offense. He attempts to shoot on partner B and take him down as many times as possible for 3 minutes. Partner B is designated as defense for round 1, and he must defend as many take down attempts as possible for 3 minutes.

➢ When the round is over, a 1-minute rest period is followed by round 2.

➢ For round 2, the partners switch so that partner A is on defense, and partner B is on offense. 1 point is scored for each successful takedown, and the winner is obviously the one with more points. Another way to rotate from offense to defense is to have the partners switch every 30 seconds so that each plays offense and defense for the 3 minute round.

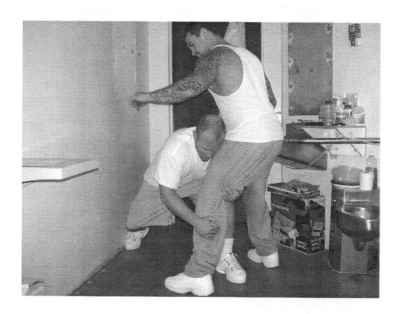

❖   3-partner take down/defend.

This is the same as take down defend except with 3 partners and a different rotation. The 3 partners stand 2 on the outside of 1 in the middle. Partner A stands on the outside facing partner B who is in the middle. Partner C stands behind partner B.

➢ For round 1, partner B shoots one time on partner A attempting to score a takedown. He then turns around and shoots on partner C once to score a take down. Partner A and partner C defend each take down attempt.

➢ For round 2, the partners rotate so that partner C is now in the middle on offense with partners A and B on the outside, and on defense.

➢ The rotations continue so that each partner is on offense in the middle, and defense on the outside. The other option is for the 3 partners starting in the same position, but partner B will first shoot on partner A, then he will turn around to defend a shoot from partner C. So the guy in the middle plays offense and defense. All partners are rotated so that they get a turn in the middle.

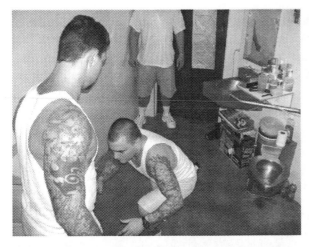 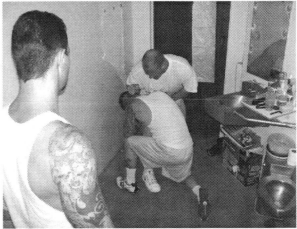

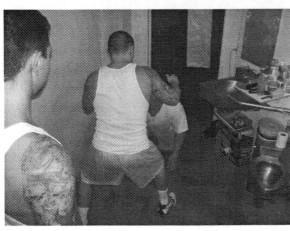 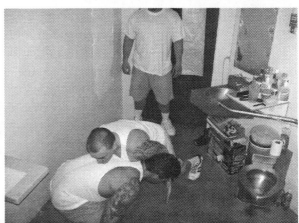

❖ **3-partner box/wrestle.**

This is the same type of drill as the 3 partner take down defend drill. The 3 partners stand in the same order (partner A outside facing partner B, partner C behind partner B.) Partners A and B have gloves or another form of wrapping on their hands.

➢ For round 1, partners A and B box for one minute.

➢ Then partner B turns around to wrestle partner C for one minute. This is repeated for a four minute round.

➢ The partners rotate positions so that each has a turn in the middle.

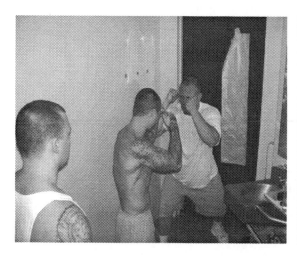 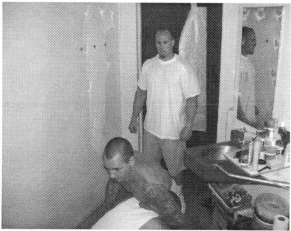

❖ **Escape from bottom/maintain top.**

This is a grappling drill that can be done with two partners, or more partners rotating every so often. For this drill, one partner starts on top of the other partner in a dominant position. His objective is to maintain that dominant position for specific time period (usually 3-5 minute rounds), and not allow the partner on bottom to escape. The partner on bottom attempts to escape. If the partner on bottom does escape, the partners return to the start position and begin again.

➢ Partner A starts in the bottom (mounted) position with partner B on top.

➢ As the round begins Partner A attempts to escape from the bottom. Partner B tries to keep his dominate position.

➢ The partners switch positions each round.

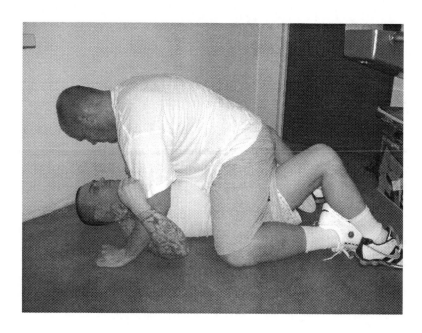

❖ Bottom to top reverse.

This drill is similar to the escape from bottom maintain top drill, except that the purpose is practice escaping only.

➢ Partner A begins on the bottom position. Partner B is on top.

➢ Partner A utilizes a technique designed specifically to escape from the bottom position to the top dominant position.

➢ Now that partner B is on bottom (mounted) position, he uses a different technique to escape the mounted position, which will bring the two partners back to the start position.

➢ This is repeated a designated number of times, or for timed rounds.

➢ The partners switch starting positions each round.

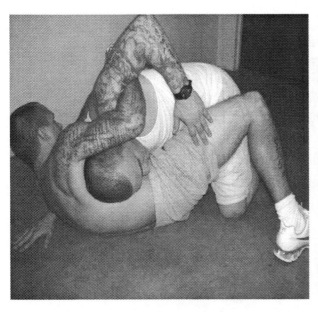 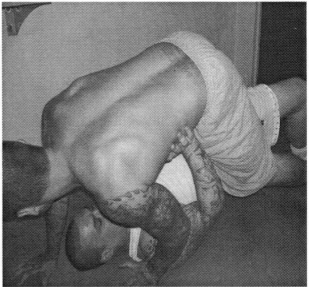

❖ Rotations.

Rotations are used when there are more than two partners. For example, when there are three partners, partners A and B will wrestle for one round. At the end of the round, partner A will rotate out, partner C will rotate in and partners B and C will wrestle for a round.

➢ Partners A and B wrestle for 1 minute.

➢ Partner A rotates out and partner C rotates in.

➢ Partners B and C wrestle for one minute.

➢ Partner B rotates out and partner A rotates in, then partners A and C wrestle. This is 1 cycle complete.

➢ Repeat. This type of rotation is also used for boxing.

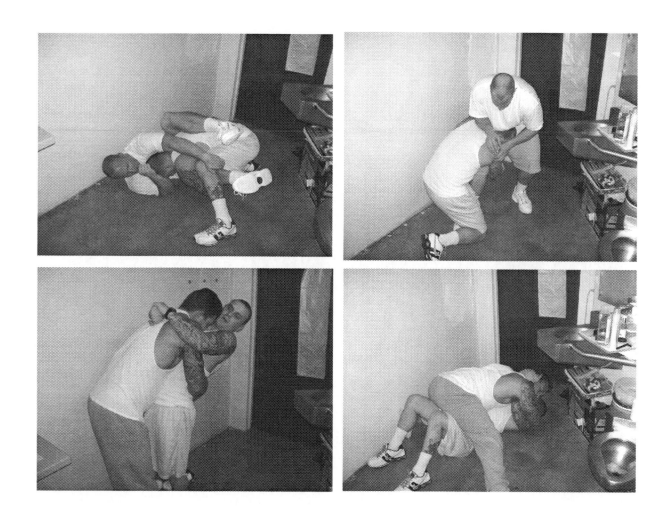

❖ Random rotation.

Random rotation is different than the regular type of rotation. Again, this drill is used when there are more than two partners. Instead of each partner getting an equal amount of active time and rest time, the rotations are at random intervals, and resemble a two against one scenario.

➢ Round 1 is partner A's round; he will wrestle partners B and C.

➢ The round begins and partner A wrestles partner B. As B begins to tire, he will tag out to partner C who is fresh. Partner C will wrestle and tag out to partner B when he gets tired. Partner A must wrestle both of the other partners for the entire round; he will get no rest. Rounds are usually 5 minutes.

➢ After a 1-2 minute rest, round 2 begins and it is partner B's round to wrestle the other two partners.

➢ Each round the partners rotate. This type of rotation is also used for boxing.

Sequence (4).

Sequences are used to practice maneuvering. These drills are performed over and over again to allow the body and mind to adapt to the movement. In this example:

➢ Partners begin by standing facing one another. Partner A then takes down partner B.

➢ After the take down, partner A moves into a dominant position.

➢ Partner A now uses a technique to submit his opponent.

➢ The partners return to the start position, and repeat.

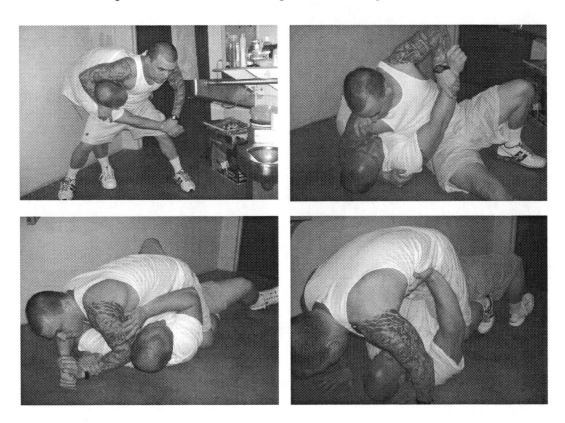

❖ Grappling/striking 100's.

Grappling and striking 100's are drills that repeat the same movement for 100 repetitions. An example of a grappling 100's, is Partner A performing 100 arm-bars on partner B. An example of striking 100's, is partner A performing 100 leg kicks on a pad held by partner B.

❖ Striking/grappling combos.

These are drills repeated as in 100's or sequences. For example, partner A will throw a 2-punch combo followed by a kick and a shoot on partner B. The partners will rotate and repeat.

Circuit Training

Circuit training is simply performing multiple exercises in succession. An example of this is performing a set of push-ups, followed by a set of squats, followed by a set of crunches to complete one cycle or circuit. Circuit training is used to save time, increase intensity, add cardio-pulmonary work, and basically get more out of your workout time. Circuit training is the core of the workouts that are demonstrated in this book, and is also the core of all of my personal workouts, and the workouts of those people that I have trained. Why? Because they work great!

Circuits can be done in a number of ways including:

- They can be done by performing one set of a certain exercise, followed by a rest period, and then followed by another exercise. Example: push-ups, rest; squats, rest; crunches, rest; repeat. In this type of circuit a rest period follows each exercise before the next exercise is performed.

- Circuits can be done at different stations or in one spot. Example: if using stations at a gym or even a public park, one would perform a set of push-ups, run over to another area and perform squats, and then run to a third area to perform crunches. In one spot the person would perform all three exercises in one area.

- Another way of performing circuits is to do the exercises continuously one after the other without rest in between each exercise. These circuits are usually done in intervals. Meaning, going back and forth from higher intensity exercises to lower intensity exercises. The reason for this is because higher intensity exercise can only be sustained for a shorter period of time. Example: 10 squat jumps, followed by 20 toe touches (standing), followed by 10 push-ups, and finally 10 jumping jacks. The squat jumps are high intensity, followed by toe touches, a lower intensity exercise. Then, push-ups are higher intensity, followed by jumping jacks, which are lower intensity.

- A fourth way of performing a circuit is to switch the exercises at a certain time during the workout. What I mean is, if a person starts out performing push-ups, squats, and crunches in succession for ten minutes, he or she will then switch to bear crawls, lunges, and supermans, for the remaining ten minutes of a twenty-minute workout.

• A fifth way of performing a circuit is to do the exercises in timed rounds with rest periods between each round. This is usually used for the more intense workouts. A simple example is a one-minute round of sprints, followed by a one-minute rest, and then a one-minute round of burpees followed by another rest etc.

Benefits of Circuit Training

There are a number of benefits to performing exercises in a circuit rather than simply doing a set of exercise followed by a rest etc.

One of the best benefits that are reaped due to performing exercises in a circuit is the cardio-pulmonary benefit. Because different parts of the body are being worked in a shorter amount of time, the heart and lungs must work harder to pump oxygen and nutrient rich blood to the different sets of muscles. For instance, when doing an upper-body exercise such as triceps extensions, the arms require oxygen rich blood, so the heart and lungs must work together to get it there. But, when an arm exercise is followed by a leg exercise, both body parts are now in need of blood flow. Therefore, the heart and lungs are worked even harder to keep the blood flowing to the two areas of the body, rather than just one area of the body. A positive side effect of this extra work done by the heart and lungs is an overall increase in endurance.

Another benefit to performing circuits is the time that is saved. Occasionally, a person will not have the time they would like to workout. In these instances circuits are great because more exercise can be done in a shorter amount of time.

Consider this scenario: A person wishes to perform ten sets of leg exercises and ten sets of core exercises, but only has twenty minutes in which to workout. Normally this person will perform one set of leg exercise followed by a one-minute rest period, to give the legs adequate time to recover. Considering the fact that it takes twenty to thirty seconds to perform each set of exercise, if the exercise periods and rest periods are multiplied by ten (because there will be ten sets and ten rest periods) the total time to perform the exercises and rest periods will be fifteen minutes. This only leaves five minutes to perform the core exercises! However, if this individual were to perform the leg and core exercises in a circuit fashion, he or she would have enough time. This is because the ten minutes that he or she would have used to rest the legs will be put to better use performing core exercises. The legs still get the rest period while the core exercises are being performed. In addition, the core muscles get a rest while the leg exercises are being performed. When performing a circuit the twenty-minute workout would look more like this: A set of leg exercise followed immediately by a set of core exercise followed by a rest period. Lets say that both the leg exercise and the core exercise take thirty seconds to perform. Performing one set of legs followed by a set of core will then take one minute. Followed by a one-minute rest. Multiply this by ten, and you get ten leg exercises and ten core exercises in twenty minutes. This is a simple example, but it helps to illustrate the timesaving benefit of circuit training.

Intensity Levels of Circuits

As I mentioned, there are different ways of performing circuits. And, like the single exercises, there are different levels of intensity that can be reached when circuit training.

One of the appealing aspects of circuits is that they can be created to reach any intensity level from very low to very high, while still reaping the benefits mentioned previously. This means that anyone at any fitness level can use and benefit from circuit training.

Intensity of exercise matters because to what extent individuals wish to take their fitness level is how high they will have to raise the intensity of exercise. In other words, in what kind of condition people want to be in is how they ought to condition themselves, or, at what level of condition a person wishes to be in, is what level of intensity the workout will have to reach. I myself use all levels of intensity to train. Some days will be very high intensity and some days will be low intensity. For my own personal use, and for this book, I have categorized three basic levels of intensity for circuits.

Rating Intensity.

For this book I will only include one way to rate intensity.

- The most obvious way to measure intensity is how hard or difficult the exercise is to perform. This is known to fitness professionals as Rating of Perceived Exertion, or RPE. Basically, how hard it feels and how much effort it takes, tells you how high the intensity is. Simple!

Increasing and Decreasing Intensity

For lowering intensity, the following strategies are used:

1. Short rest periods are included between each main exercise.

2. Lower intensity exercises are added between each main exercise, such as; standing toe touches, standing twists, or jogging lightly in place.

3. Lower intensity type exercises are used for the main exercises. For example, instead of using a jumping exercise for the lower body, a lesser intensity exercise like bodyweight squats is used.

4. The circuit is performed at a slower pace. Rather than going all-out, a pace at 50% of maximum effort is used, for example.

For increasing intensity, the following strategies are used:

1.   The main exercises are performed with reduced rest periods, or without any rest in between.

2.   Less and sometimes no lower intensity movements are included in the circuit.

3.   Higher intensity type exercises are used for the main exercises rather than lower intensity exercises. For example, instead of regular push-ups for the upper body exercise, 1 and 1 plyometric push-ups are used.

4.   The circuit is done at a faster pace. At say 65% maximal effort or higher.

Putting Circuits Together

When circuits are put together there are some things taken into consideration.

1.   What intensity level the circuit will reach.

2.   How much time the workout will take.

3.   What kind of circuit will it be (stations, one spot, interval, etc.)?

4.   Will the circuit be a whole body workout or focus on a specific region.

5.   Will the circuit be general, or have a focus such as, focus on power, endurance, or strength?

Really the sky is the limit when creating circuits. Any combination of exercises and techniques can be used to create a workout.

The point of the following circuits is to give the whole body a workout that includes resistance exercises and a cardio-respiratory benefit at the same time. In order to work the whole body the most basic circuit will utilize at least three main exercises, one exercise for the upper, one exercise for the middle, and one exercise for the lower regions of the body.

Circuits can also be created to add more emphasis to a specific region of the body. One way that this is accomplished is to make every other exercise focus on that region. For instance, if a person wanted to really focus on the core, then every other exercise in the circuit would be a core exercise. For example: Sit-ups (core); Squats; Crunches (core); Push-ups; Leg raise (core).

Example Circuits

These are some simple examples of circuits. Remember that any exercises can be used, any number of exercises can be used, and any techniques for performing exercises can be used in creating circuits for the improvement of general fitness levels. These are just simple illustrations.

Each person is different, so what one person may consider high or low intensity may be different according to another person.

The circuits are performed by completing 10-20 repetitions of each exercise before moving on to the subsequent exercise. Once the last exercise in the circuit is completed, the circuit is repeated from the beginning.

LEVEL 1 Circuits

These circuits:

➢ Utilize lower intensity exercises.

➢ Include rest periods.

➢ Are performed at a slower pace.

1. Jumping Jack—rest; Toe-touch (standing)—rest; Knee-up (standing)—rest; Squat—rest; Push-up—rest.

➢ This level 1 circuit utilizes lower intensity exercises along with rests in between each one. This circuit can be done for ten sets, meaning ten times all of the way through. Or it can be done for a specific time period such as twenty minutes. To adjust the intensity, the previous listed strategies are used.

2. 1¼ Squat—rest; Crunch—rest; 1¼ Push-up—rest.

➢ A simpler circuit, this one would actually probably be harder than the first for most people as the exercises are a little more difficult. It is still level 1 because it is done at a slower pace and with rest periods. This can easily become a level 2 circuit by reducing the rest periods though. To adjust the intensity, the previous listed strategies are used.

3. 1,2,3 Squat; Hamstring reach—rest; Windmill; Ankle reach—rest; Knee-up (standing); Push-up—rest.

➢ This circuit raises the intensity by performing two exercises between rest periods. To adjust the intensity, the previous listed strategies are used.

LEVEL 2 Circuits

These circuits:

➢ Include exercises of higher intensity.

➢ Include lower intensity exercises as the rest periods.

➢ Are done at a medium pace.

1. Lunge; Jumping Jack; Reverse crunch; Toe touch; Push-up—rest.

➢ Only one rest is included at the end of the cycle. The other "rest periods" are the Jumping jacks and Toe-touch (standing) exercises. These are lower intensity exercises so they are considered rest. To adjust the intensity up or down the previous strategies are used.

2. Pull-ups; Split squat; Duck walk; Jumping jack; Toe touch (standing); Push-ups; Windmill.

➢ Here is a good example of intervals being used. There are periods of higher intensity (going straight from pull-ups to split squats and then to duck walks) with lower intensity periods (jumping jacks and toe touches) serving as a rest. To adjust the intensity up or down the previous strategies are used.

3. Step-ups; Push-ups; Jumping jacks; Sit-up hip-up; Windmill; Bear crawl.

➢ Again intervals are plain to see as the circuit starts off with two higher intensity exercises then mixes in lower intensity periods in order to rest. To adjust the intensity up or down the previous strategies are used.

LEVEL 3 Circuits

These circuits:

➢ Include exercises of the highest intensity.

➢ Are done at a fast pace.

➢ These circuits are level 3 for a reason; they are hard!

1.   Hop-up Pull-up; Hanging knee-up; Walking piggyback squat; 1 and 1 push-up; Sprawl/sit through.

➤   To adjust intensity up or down the previous listed strategies are used.

2.   Quick step-ups; Body Hop push-ups; Pike; Bear crawl push-ups; Superman; Lunge.

➤   To adjust intensity up or down the previous listed strategies are used.

3.   Jump and tuck knees; Jumping Jacks; Jump up to push-ups; Toe touch (standing); Plyometric Pull-ups.

You can clearly see here that intervals were used. Every other exercise uses jumping techniques that are extremely hard to continually perform. These are used to increase power. The low intensity exercises between each of the harder exercises give the body time to recover and perform the next set of hard exercise, and yet keep the body moving, therefore increasing the intensity, and endurance component.

These are some simple examples of general circuits of varying intensity levels. The only limiting factor to creating circuits is the imagination.

Creating circuits with a focus.

I pointed out in the single exercises section that I, on some days, train for specific components of fitness such as strength, power, or endurance. This is because, while using the previous types of circuits for general purposes, if one really wants to improve specific components of fitness, he or she must train accordingly. To create a circuit that focuses on one component of fitness, I use the following guidelines:

Circuits that focus on strength:

1.   Include rest periods.

2.   Include exercises with added resistance, usually in the form of a partner adding resistance.

3.   Use a lower number of repetitions.

Example: Squats (with partner on shoulders)—rest; **Handstand shoulder press**—rest; **Pick-ups**—rest; **Hanging knee raise**—rest.

Circuits that focus on power:

1.   Include longer rest periods. (Unless the focus is power endurance.)

2.   Include plyometrics (jump training) exercises.

3.   Use lower number of repetitions.

Example: Jump and tuck knees—rest; **Body Hops**—rest; **Jump over object**—rest; **Clap push-ups**—rest;

Circuits that focus on endurance:

1.   Use short or no rest periods.

2.   Use high repetitions.

3.   May include added resistance exercises or plyometrics.

Example: Bear crawl push-ups; 1,2,3 Squats; Lying toe touches; Side bends; Stagger push-ups; Lunges.

Again, these are simple examples but illustrate the focus on strength exercises, power exercises, and endurance exercises.

Hardcore

This section includes examples of exercises that very few individuals actually perform. These routines are Hardcore! I don't recommend that anyone try any of these! As a matter of fact, please don't try these.

These routines are definitely high-intensity workouts and can really wear the body out. All of these circuits focus on endurance of the highest level. Most of the time they are only performed once a week, and twice a week at the most, to prevent over training.

I always perform a thorough warm-up before attempting this level of exercise. First, to prevent injuries. Second, to allow my body to get ready. And finally, so I won't vomit. Even the most in-shape individuals occasionally dry-heave when doing these routines at the correct pace.

What makes these routines so brutal is the all-out pace at which they are done. Each is done at an all-out 100% effort for the entire duration. No rest, and no intervals are used; it's all-out maximum effort for the duration of each set.

The Hardcore Routines

❖ **10 Step-ups; 10 Clap Push-ups; 10 Plyometric step-ups; 10 Push-ups.**

➢ This is one of my favorite high intensity circuits. It is also the easiest of the five routines listed here. It looks simple, but at the pace I usually do it (One cycle every 1 minute for 10-15 minutes; and slowing to one cycle every 1½ minutes, for the remaining 30-35 minutes, non-stop and no rest) it gets my heart rate up to between 180-190bpm for the 45 minute set. What makes it hard (for me anyway) is the plyometric push-ups, they really get the heart pumping. Some times I use claps, sometimes I use stagger switch etc. for the plyometric push-ups.

❖ **Pick-up; Plyo-Burpee. (Requires a partner)**

➢ This one is devastating, especially when it's done in longer rounds. It starts with partner A and partner B facing each other. Partner A picks up partner B grabbing him around his upper legs, and carries him five feet. He then sets him down and immediately drops down performing a burpee with a clap push-up. He then gets up immediately and picks partner B up and carries him another five feet before performing another plyo-burpee. This is repeated non-stop and without any rest period. Usually this one is done in rounds of 1-5 minutes. No stopping; no slowing down.

❖ **Leg drive; Push-up; Pick-up. (Requires a partner)**

➢ This one is another killer. Partners A and B stand facing each other. Partner A then leg drives Partner B for ten full seconds. Partner B uses all of his strength to stop partner A's progress. Once the ten seconds is up, partner A drops down and performs a push-up. He then gets up and picks up partner B to carry him back to the starting point. This is done in either timed rounds of 1-5 minutes or sets of 5-10. No stopping; no slowing down.

❖ **Sprint; Plyo push-up.**

➢ Simple but vicious, this routine is done by sprinting for approximately 25 yards, turning around, and sprinting back. Once back at the starting point, 20, 1 and 1 push-ups are performed. Immediately the cycle is repeated. For the push-ups, the descending reps technique is used so that the next time only 19, 18, 17 etc. are performed. This is repeated non-stop, sprinting down and back and completing the descending set of push-ups, for 5-minute rounds. The sprints will begin to slow down and become very unpleasant, while the push-ups will begin to feel like a welcomed rest period!

❖ **Heavy bag; Jump; plyo push-up.**

➢ This is another of my favorites. Partner A stands facing a heavy bag that partner B is holding. Partner B holds a watch as well as he will have to yell out "go" every 15 seconds to partner A. It starts when Partner B says, "go". Partner A immediately performs a jump up and tuck knees to chest jump. Upon landing, he drops straight down and performs a clap push-up. He now pops back up and hits the bag left, right, left, right as fast and hard as he possibly can. He never stops except for when partner B yells out "go". When partner B does yell out 'go", he performs the two jumping exercises. This happens every 15 seconds. This is done for 5-minute rounds.

Works Consulted

Hatfield, Fredrick C. Ph.D. *Fitness The Complete Guide.* 8.1.5 ed. International Sports Sciences Association, 2004.

Bryant, Cedric X., Ph.D., and Daniel J. Green. *ACE Personal Trainer Manual.* 3rd ed. American Council on Exercise, 2003

Bompa, Tudor O. Ph.D., and Michael C. Carrera. *Periodization Training for Sports.* 2nd ed. Human Kinetics, 2005

Chu, Donald A. Ph.D. *Jumping Into Plyometrics.* 2nd ed. Human Kinetics, 1998

Brooks, Douglas S. MS. *Program Design for Personal Trainers.* Mammoth Lakes, California: Moves International, 2004

About the Author

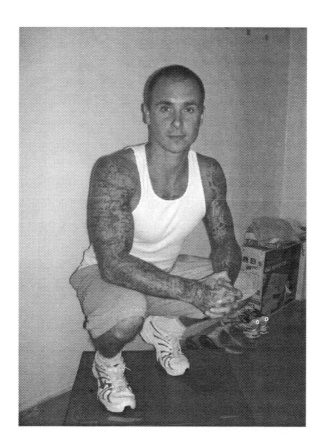

Steven Hansen is the founder of Get Serious Fitness. He is a Certified Personal Trainer, and an active member of both The American Council on Exercise, and The International Sports Sciences Association. He continues his studies in the fields of fitness and business. To find out more about the author or the individuals who appear in this book go to: www.Myspace.com/getseriouseriousfitness.

To contact the author, send E-mail to:

www.getseriousfitness@Yahoo.com